FARMCARTS

A History of the Military

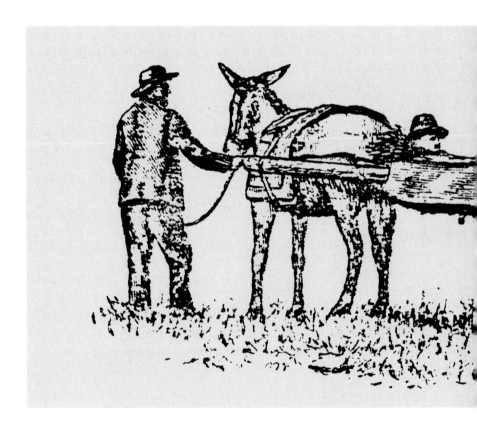

SOUTHERN ILLINOIS UNIVERSITY PRESS •
• Carbondale and Edwardsville

TO FORDS

Ambulance, 1790–1925

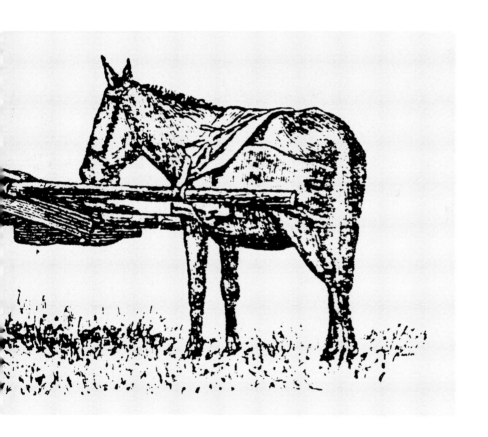

JOHN S. HALLER, JR.

Library of Congress Cataloging-in-Publication Data

Haller, John S.
    Farmcarts to Fords: a history of the military ambulance, 1790–1925 / John S.
Haller, Jr.
      p.   cm. — (Medical humanities series)
    Includes bibliographical references and index.
    1. Transport of sick and wounded—History.   2. Transportation, Military—
History. 3. Ambulances—History. I. Title. II. Series.
    [DNLM: 1. Ambulances—history. 2. Military Medicine—history.
3. Transportation of Patients—history. 500 H185f]
UH500.H35 1992
355.3′45—dc20
DNLM/DLC
for Library of Congress   92-3772
ISBN 0-8093-1817-2   CIP

No spectacle is more painful than that of the carriage of the wounded, the sick, and the dying in the midst of a campaign. It is the blackest page of war. The triumphs of the battlefield are all dimmed in looking at this inevitable sequel. It is needful to have seen it to comprehend it, for official dispatches and history tell but little of the reality.

—Sir Henry Holland,
Recollections of Past Life, 1872

Contents

Plates

Acknowledgments

During the course of writing this book, many colleagues, librarians, archivists, and friends provided support, suggestions, criticism, and encouragement. In this regard, I am especially indebted to David L. Wilson, colleague in the Department of History; to Pascal James Imperato, M.D., at the Medical Society for the State of New York and editor of the *New York State Journal of Medicine*; and to Glen W. Davidson, chair of the Department of Medical Humanities at the Southern Illinois University School of Medicine in Springfield, for their timely counsel, suggestions, and assistance. Also important are those reviewers whose evaluations—both supportive and critical—caused me to adjust my sights, correct mistakes, clarify concepts, and explore new areas and connections. For their comments I am deeply appreciative. I want to give special thanks to Richard D. DeBacher, editorial director of Southern Illinois University Press, for his advocacy on behalf of the manuscript; and to Susan Wilson and Kathryn Koldehoff, whose editorial support added measurably to the final product. In addition, I appreciate the encouragement and advice given by colleagues Mark S. Foster, David P. Werlich, Donald S. Detwiler, John Y. Simon, Robert L. Hohlfelder, Glendon F. Drake, Gilbert Schmidt, David C. Hood, Thomas J. Noel, Mary S. Conroy, Dorothy Abrahamse, Stephen Horn, Karen Fawson, and Barbara Parker. Finally, I should like to thank my wife, Robin, who, as with all of my research, offered inspiration, encouragement, criticism, and substantial assistance, including the proofing of numerous drafts and indexing the finished manuscript.

Like most authors of historical works, I am especially obligated to the historian-collector-librarians and their professional staffs. It was their generosity of time and experienced assistance that made it possible for me to enrich my understanding of the subject matter and to carry out the necessary research. These individuals include Patricia Breivik, Jordan M. Scepanski, James F. Williams, Kathy Fahey, George W. Black, Kenneth G. Peterson, Lori Arp, Elnora M. Mercado, Betsy Porter, Jay Schafer, Connie Whitson, Mary Lou Goodyear, Rutherford Witthus, Eveline L. Yang, Joan Fiscella, Jean Hemphill, Marilyn Mitchell, and Muriel E. Woods. Finally, my gratitude would not be complete without noting the fine libraries whose collections I used. These include Morris Library of Southern Illinois University at Carbondale; California State University, Long Beach Library; the Norlin and Auraria Libraries of the University of Colorado; Denison Memorial Library of the University of Colorado Health Sciences Center; Infantry School Library at Fort Benning; Clemson College Library; Matthews Library of Arizona State; Oregon Health Science University Library; Southwestern Presbyterian University Library; University of Washington Library; University of California at San Diego; Lane Medical Library of Stanford University; John Crerar Library of the University of Chicago; University of South Carolina Libraries; Linscheid Library of East Central University; University of California at Irvine; Kansas State Library; University of Illinois Library; University of Arizona Library; Medical Library of the University of Missouri; United States Air Force Academy Library; Harold B. Lee Library of Brigham Young University; University of Denver Library; Moody Memorial Library of Baylor University; Creighton University Health Sciences Library; Aurora Public Library in Colorado; Rudolph Matas Medical Library of Tulane University; Enoch Pratt Free Library of Baltimore; Vanderbilt University Medical Center Library; New York Academy of Medicine Library; University of California at Los Angeles — Bio-Medical Library; University of Minnesota — Bio-Medical Library; Boston Public Library; Newberry Library; the Library of Congress; and the National Library of Medicine.

Farmcarts to Fords

Introduction

The word *ambulance*, from the Latin *ambulare*, meaning to walk or move from place to place, was applied to the French *hôpital ambulant* by Surgeon Dominique-Jean Larrey during the Napoleonic Wars. Larrey referred to "temporary hospital establishments, organized near the divisions of an army, to follow their movements and to assure early succor to the wounded." He and later Europeans included wagons, drivers, surgeons, supplies, and all material support within the meaning of the term.[1]

Decades later, British Surgeon General Thomas Longmore explained in the ninth edition of the *Encyclopaedia Britannica* (1875) that ambulances, in military parlance, were "hospital establishments moving with armies in the field, and organized for providing early surgical assistance to the wounded after battles." His definition differed little from that provided by Larrey. Essentially, ambulances were intended to provide temporary assistance to the wounded, thus distinguishing them from stationary or fixed hospitals, where the sick and wounded received care and treatment "of a more permanent character." Nevertheless, according to Longmore, the term *ambulance* in American and British usage was frequently misapplied to the two- or four-wheeled "ambulance wagon" or wheeled-transport conveyance, which carried wounded from the battlefield to

1

temporary and fixed hospitals. Thus, while the term *six ambulances* typically referred to six field hospitals attached to the army and moving with it, in England and America it also meant six wagons.[2] As late as 1909, Lieutenant Colonel William G. Macpherson, writing in the *Journal of the Royal Army Medical Corps* on medical support and organization, warned against calling an ambulance wagon an ambulance. For him, an ambulance was "a mobile medical unit, and it must be used to express the unit only." Notwithstanding this intent, the British and American corruption of the word, growing out of the experiences and language of the Crimean and American Civil wars, confused usage to the extent that both meanings have prevailed into the present day. In this book, I trace both histories, from their origin, through the Great War, and into its aftermath.[3]

Any study of the ambulance, however defined, cannot be viewed apart from military science, military hygiene and sanitation, military surgery, and military-medical administration. The effects of technology and organization on the moving and supplying of armies; changes in military strategy from close-order volley firing in linear platoons to artillery and open-order skirmishes; the development of breech-loading rifled cannon, high-velocity small arms, explosive shells, shrapnel, hand grenades, and bombs; and the introduction of railroads challenged the very assumptions on which planners built their medical evacuation systems. The same proved true of motorized vehicles and of offensive measures, such as gas attacks and air raids.

Timely and effective evacuation of wounded not only avoided the permanent loss of a soldier's services but maintained the morale of those who remained to fight. Clearly, when soldiers faced the prospect of abandonment by their officers and comrades, they were less willing to fight. In addition, it eliminated the likelihood that able-bodies soldiers would leave the firing line to assist wounded comrades to safety. The presence of hospitals near the field of battle also reflected an intent by the military to return the wounded soldier to his unit as quickly as possible. In other words, the farther back the wounded were evacuated, the less likely they were to return to their units. Finally, an efficient system of medical evacuation maintained morale on the home front.

The time available to collect, treat, and distribute wounded soldiers to appropriate medical facilities weighed heavily as medical planners sought to adjust their evacuation systems to new strategies and technologies, to wars of movement versus stationary wars, and to the competing needs of replacement troops and matériel that demanded access to the same roads and transport. Each battle had its own set of dynamics and its own decision points: whether to collect the more seriously wounded first or to leave them to the enemy during retreat; whether to risk ambulance bearers in open engagements, when improved weaponry made them more vulnerable, or to leave the casualties to collect in "nests" until night or a lull in the battle; whether to risk doctors and surgeons close to the front line in a stationary war or to rely on an efficient transport system to convey the wounded to ambulance stations further to the rear; whether to treat gunshot wounds and fractures on the basis of aseptic treatment or to consider every wound infected. As history has shown, the answers often meant the difference between well-ordered, life-preserving relief to the wounded and demoralizing debacles that wasted lives and destroyed armies and nations. Paul Bronsart von Schellendorff (1832–91) remarked in his *Duties of the General Staff* (1895) that "the system of evacuating sick forms the basis of the entire medical service in the field." Like links in a chain, the failure of one link nullified the ability of the others to perform their functions. When the system failed, for whatever reason, the military faced the harshness of public condemnation.[4]

I have chosen to give greater emphasis to the development of British and American evacuation procedures and technology than to those of other nations. Notwithstanding this preference, this history is a seam within a much broader cloth. This has meant drawing broad comparisons and contrasts, looking for elements of continuity from one war or nation to another, and demonstrating common problems. The interested reader should also understand that, while a number of different wars are included in this study, my intent has not been to cover all aspects of medical evacuation or, for that matter, to give equal treatment to all developments. To do so would have required writing several books or expanding the present study beyond what I had originally intended. For that reason, hospital ships are treated more peripherally than are hand conveyances, wheeled vehicles, and other types of ground transportation. The emphasis on immediate ground transportation and medical evacuation systems highlights the common dilemmas that faced the victorious and the defeated on the battlefield, the revolutionary challenges to the old order, the irksome internal conflicts confronting planners and sanitarians, the impact of new technology, and the persistence of old problems in new situations. By focusing primarily on hand conveyances and wheeled vehicles, I have been able to recount with greater force and clarity what, for many nations and their armies, were common problems, incongruities, and acknowledged controversies. All too often, the sick and wounded were sacrificed to a military Moloch without reason, without intelligence, and without compassion. Yet, along with the martial chorus that heralded the beginnings of the modern Leviathan state, there was also born a desire to bring help and dignity to the sick and wounded in war.

PART ONE

Early History

1

Beginnings of a System

Although history burgeons with stories of battles fought, victories won, and warriors' triumphs, seldom does it follow the course of those who dropped out of battle with sickness or with wounds. Nevertheless, their story is worth telling for it represents the underside of war, explaining the grim lot of the sick or wounded soldier and an army's commitment—in victory or defeat—to its fighting forces. Until most recent times, armies commonly suffered high mortality and morbidity from faulty sanitation and disease: diarrhea and dysentery, respiratory diseases, skin infections, smallpox, scurvy, measles, typhus fever, yellow fever, diphtheria, whooping cough, and influenza. There was little need to succor the wounded since during the battle, or afterwards, the victors preferred to massacre the enemy's wounded and treat their own with indifference. The more fortunate were carried to the rear by comrades. Most, however, were left to lie exposed until after the battle, and surgical assistance, if any, did not reach them until a day or more after the engagement. Then, the wounded received aid from servants, camp followers, wives, bandsmen, and local inhabitants, who moved about the field in search of the living and available booty.

EARLY MANAGEMENT SYSTEMS

Improved management systems, beginning as early as 1200 B.C. in Egypt, encouraged governments to recognize the economy of saving the lives of career soldiers, who represented a costly investment in a state's military armamentaria. After a victorious battle against the Etruscans in 480 B.C., Roman consul Manlius billeted wounded soldiers (including enemy soldiers) in private homes until their wounds healed. On the frontiers of the Roman empire, a system of medical care developed in the first and second centuries A.D. known as *valetudinaria*, which consisted of single rows of rooms built around a rectangular courtyard. Designed originally by Roman landlords as sick quarters for their slaves, the *valetudinaria* eventually evolved to include the care of the sick and wounded soldier.

Under the empire, a regular medical corps served the Roman army and navy, the most famous of whom was Dioscorides, a native of Cilicia (Turkey), who served the army during the reign of Nero (A.D. 54–68). Foreign medics within the Roman army treated the wounded on the field of battle, as well as in military hospitals. Field generals placed the legionary in the care of *medicus ordinarius, medicus cohortis*, and *medicus legionis* who, while acting as soldiers first, provided the basis of medical care on the field and in the *valetudinaria*. The *medici* did not so much constitute a separate medical corps as they provided a combination of soldiery and care.[1]

Although armies from Alexander the Great to the Romans had taken prisoners rather than having killed them (since they made good slaves), later armies found little use in this humanitarian gesture. For the wounded soldier, probably the best that could happen was to be killed outright rather than face the prospect of medical indifference in the hands of his own colleagues or a parting sword thrust from the enemy as he left the field following the battle. At the defense of Metz (October 20 to December 26, 1552) and the subsequent siege of Thérouanne in 1553, however, the Spanish army chose to save its prisoners; afterwards, the customary practice of slaughtering unransomed prisoners declined.[2]

While armies continued to experience hand-to-hand encounters, the technology of warfare and the extended range of weaponry resulted in battle wounds of a more impersonal nature. This, plus the occasional spirit of humanity, sometimes inhibited the gruesome practice of killing off the wounded. Nonetheless, armies left their wounded exposed until the fighting ceased, except, if circumstances allowed, when they could assist them to the rear. Physicians and surgeons accompanied armies on their campaigns, treating the wounded, even providing care stations for convalescents. However, surgeons generally served the ranking officers, not the common soldier, whose only support was the ditch where he fell or the occasional barber-surgeon, wandering empiric, bonesetter, tooth puller, or charlatan, who attended to his wounds. In any case, surgical assistance became available only after battle. In certain periods, a victorious army placed care of its sick and wounded enemy in the hands of local populations, who then demanded ransom for their return. Although seemingly insensitive, this practice assured a modicum of care to the wounded soldier because of his future value.[3]

The earliest known written records of wars also comment on transportation for the sick and wounded. Indeed, the work of the ambulance bearer is probably coextensive with the history of mankind, being described as early as 1000 B.C. in the *Iliad* of Homer.[4] Examples in oral and written history cross boundaries; in western Europe, ambulance support existed among the Anglo-Saxons, Normans, and English as early as A.D. 900 and probably long before then. Not until the fifteenth century, however, did there appear in military organization a unit equipped specifically to provide both transport and emergency treatment of sick and wounded.[5]

During the Crusades, which historians have sometimes likened to little more than "undisciplined caravans," the wounded were carried on litters suspended between two horses, using the long triangular shield of the Crusader as a stretcher. A number of knightly orders, including the Knights Hospitallers, or Knights of St. John, and the Teutonic Knights, aided pilgrims and nursed the sick. The Knights of St. John (1211) subsequently became the Knights of Rhodes (1311) and the Knights of Malta (1530). The Germans in 1143 established the Teutonic Knights of St. Mary's Hospital in Jerusalem; eventually this teutonic order expanded its influence throughout Prussia.[6]

With the establishment of large, standing armies of mercenary troops, the number of medical personnel increased considerably to meet the needs of the new rank and file. This support for the wounded was especially evident in the armies of Charles VII of France (r. 1422–61) and Maximilian I of Germany (1459–1519), in the wars of the Swiss Confederation (1315–1798), and with the work of such physicians as Colnet and Morestede at Agincourt (1415), Gabriel Miron at Naples (1494), Marcello Cumano with the Milanese at Novara (1513), and Louis Desbourges at Pavia (1525). During these wars, state monies paid "field barbers" to accompany troops and attend the wounded after battle, provide bandaging material, support nontransportable wounded at improvised hospitals, underwrite expenses of wagon transportation, and even send convalescents to mineral baths. Still, little was done to support the wounded until the conclusion of battle.[7]

A physician and surgeon accompanied Edward III (r. 1326–77) in war; and, during Henry V's (r. 1413–22) campaign of the Somme in 1415, the king purchased medical stores for his twenty-five hundred men-at-arms and eight thousand archers. Since Henry had no wheeled transport, the wounded presumably found their own transportation, probably commandeering country carts from neighboring farms.[8]

Queen Isabella I of Spain was the first European monarch to authorize organized support for the wounded in battle. At the siege of Álora (1484) and of Baza (1489), during the conquest of Granada, and during the expulsion of the Moors, the Spanish army employed wagons with beds to carry the wounded from the battle lines to large hospital tents. Transport wagons and field hospitals (*ambulancias*) were also used during the siege of Otrera (1477–78) and the capture of Málaga (August 19, 1487). The Queen's Hospital, comprising six tents and equipment, physicians, surgeons, attendants, and nearly four hundred wagons, was her gift to her army in war. Isabella's grandson Charles V (r. 1519–56) followed her example by deploying the sick and wounded to the baggage train and to field tents, where they were attended by physicians and barber-surgeons and nursed by female camp followers.[9]

In France, Charles the Bold (1433–77) attached a surgeon to every company of one hundred lancers and provided his court with six physicians, four surgeons, and forty assistants to attend wounds incurred in battle or at tournaments. By the time of the siege of Amiens (1597) in the reign of Henry IV (1589–1610), France had established stationary military hospitals, supported by ambulance service and first aid. Despite these humanitarian approaches, however, most field commanders considered battle casualties a continual nuisance that impeded the movements of the army. Few were willing to digress from their battle plans in order to provide for their needs. For that reason, armies gave little more than lip service to medical support—a neglect that proved fatal to many of the injured.[10]

War surgery underwent significant changes in the sixteenth century, following the development of the wheel lock (1515) in small firearms. Accompanying this innovation, such surgeons as Hans von Gersdorff, Hieronymus Brunschwig (1450–1533), Giovanni da Vigo (1460–1520), and Paracelsus (1493–1541) contributed to both the theory and practice of treating gunshot wounds. The greatest European military surgeon, Ambroise Paré (1510–90), lived through the reigns of seven French monarchs and divided his skills between military surgery in the French army and private practice in Paris. Paré made his reputation as a skilled surgeon following his experiences with Francis I in Turin in 1536–37. His introduction of the ligature in amputation represented a major innovation in surgery, replacing the earlier practice of cauterization by boiling oil or water and heated cautery. Paré also invented several surgical instruments, developed artificial limbs and eyes, suspected flies as carriers of wound infections, experimented with trusses and teeth implantations, and challenged the popular belief that gunshot wounds were poisoned.[11]

The establishment of camp and stationary hospitals and homes for disabled soldiers (*maisons des invalides*) accompanied the military surgeon. The first permanent military hospital was the Hôtel Royal des Invalides, founded by Louis XIV in 1674, followed by the English military hospital at Chelsea in 1682. During this same period, barber-surgeons were assigned as medical personnel in times of war. Elector George Wilhelm (1619–40) of Brandenburg provided a barber for every regiment and a field barber for every company of infantry and cavalry. And in 1708, Louis XIV directed hospital personnel consisting of two hundred physicians and surgeons to attend the needs of sick and wounded officers and soldiers. In addition, the French erected some fifty-one military hospitals in their cities, with specific directions and regulations governing the duties of hospital personnel and medical treatment of patients. By the mid-eighteenth century, most of Europe's armies had clearly defined medical services, as well as regulations establishing and governing the different forms of fixed and ambulant hospitals.[12]

Also by the eighteenth century, military medicine had become largely the function of government and, consequently, involved medical examination of recruits, military regulation of army hospitals, and publication of printed orders and bulletins devoted to hygiene. During the course of the century's wars, armies established stationary as well as field hospitals and dressing stations at the rear of fighting columns and even designated detachments responsible for evacuation of the wounded. Following the battle of Liegnitz during the Seven Years' War, Frederick the Great ordered five hundred dragoons to dismount and give saddle transportation to the wounded. On the field of Kunersdorf (1759), he ordered the bandaging of wounded during the battle. Similarly, during and after the battle of Fontenoy (1745), Francis Boucher reported that regimental surgeons performed amputations on the battlefield, carried out operations at ambulance stations behind the lines, and evacuated the wounded by caissons and carts to civilian hospitals, churches, and private homes in Lille and Donai some sixteen to twenty miles from the battlefield.[13]

PRUSSIAN TACTICS

Both the desire and the ability to evacuate wounded during battle is determined in large measure by the nature of the terrain, the condition of roads, the nature of the battle, the kinds of weapons used, the state of technology, and the state of the art of medicine. For the eighteenth century, the determining factors were the tactics of Frederick the Great (1712–86), who deployed his troops for both attack and defense in long thin lines of foot and light forces, with cavalry standing on the flanks or in the rear. Each battalion had a gun or more and, at certain points in the line, batteries of reserve heavy caliber. Battles opened with artillery, followed by the first line of attackers advancing within musket range (150–200 yards) and attempting to break down the opposite side with its fire-by-file, followed by a bayonet charge. During this time, the cavalry attempted to outflank and attack the enemy's foot troops. Tactics included advancing and retiring in line, wheelings, ployments and deployments, and forward and flank marches in close or open column. Perhaps Frederick's greatest contribution to military tactics was his attention to mobility on the battlefield, especially his desire for a successful flank attack.[14]

The unreliability and inaccuracy of the flintlock musket required certain compensations in battle tactics, including mass fire from elongated lines, which were three-deep, parade-style precision movements that ensured accurate distance and alignments, and the heavy reliance on cavalry and artillery to disrupt the deployment of the enemy's forces. Historian Theodore A. Dodge described the tactics accordingly:

> Concentric attacks were common, in front and on the flanks and rear of the enemy's army; but unless these attacks could be timed so as smartly to work together, the result was apt to be failure. The army acting on the defensive fought in place after much the same fashion, relying on its artillery and infantry fire; and the second line and cavalry assisted the first line. The retiring of the first line was wont to have an ill effect on the second. Hence, unless the first line of the army on the defensive could stand off the enemy's first line and cavalry to good effect, this army would be apt, for fear of defeat, to break off the battle and retire to a fresh field, an operation . . . of slow maneuvre much more easy of accomplishment . . . as the opponent was rarely ready to follow.[15]

Frederick's tactics precipitated a host of imitators, and, by the 1770s, Prussian precision in drill and execution had become incorporated in the regulations of most European armies. Nevertheless, much of this would change as a result of light-infantry deployment in the Seven Years' War and the lessons learned during the American War of Independence.

During the years of America's struggles, the organization of permanent divisions, the use of individual fire, the reintroduction of skirmishers, and the vulnerability of linear tactics to the open-order fighting of undisciplined marksmen became harsh lessons to be learned by England's armies. They also became the basis of thoughtful new tactics brought home by French soldiers fighting in the colonies and eventually incorporated into the military tactics of the patriotic forces during the French Revolution. There, patriotic fervor combined with a system of light troops as skirmishers fought in open order, backed by battalion columns attacking with bayonet. Covered by artillery fire and sustained by cavalry, these troops brought an end to Frederick's tactical dominance. First Baron de Mésnil-Durand, then Joly de Maizeroy and François Philippe de Bohan challenged Frederick's system of long and rigid lines. Although the Prussian system remained in force until the Ordinance of 1791, it was all but dormant during the Republic and the Empire. Except for parade movements and defensive operations, the Prussian system gave way to the French formation in which skirmishers kept up a constant curtain of fire and movement to conceal the deployment of columns as they advanced to charging distance. Napoléon would perfect this formation into a fine martial art, followed by its incorporation into the French Regulations of 1831 and Prussian Regulations of 1847.[16]

THE FRENCH SYSTEM

Although the roots of the ambulance as a mobile medical unit can be found in the artifacts of earlier centuries, it is basically a modern concept derived principally from changes in late-eighteenth- and early-nineteenth-century military tactics, innovations in surgery, and the design of lighter field transport. The first perceptible change in medical evacuation systems occurred in the French army of the Rhine under the command of General Adam-Philippe de Custine (1740–93). There, a young military surgeon, Dominique-Jean Larrey (1766–1842), from Beaudeau in the Pyrénées, demonstrated that a more responsive arrangement for the removal of the wounded could save valuable troops. Larrey joined the Army of the Rhine in 1792 (meeting Napoléon at Toulon in 1794) and took part in sixty battles and four hundred engagements. Devoting a lifetime to military surgery, he improved wound excision, developed a semicircular surgical needle with a lancet-shaped cutting point, avoided ointments and greases in dressing wounds, and used warm camphorated wine or Labarraque's solution in washing wounds. Although noteworthy as a military surgeon, Larrey's greatest contributions were his medical evacuation procedures and his administration.[17]

Larrey was appointed medical chief of a division of the Army of the Rhine just thirteen months prior to the Reign of Terror. At that time, the sick and wounded customarily collected at the baggage train in the rear of the battle zone, where surgeons, supported by cumbersome *fourgons* drawn by forty or more horses, attended to those soldiers able to walk or to those who were carried the distance. Because of their size and the confusion of battle, few of the *fourgons* reached the actual scene of battle until twenty-four or thirty-six hours after the engagement. All too often, those soldiers unable to leave the firing line because of their wounds died of shock or loss of blood before medical support arrived.

Larrey did not invent ambulant hospitals (Queen Isabella I of Spain had introduced them as early as 1487); rather, he provided the existing hospital with an effective form of light transportation. His idea was to follow the advanced guard in much the same manner as did the "flying artillery" (*artillerie volant*) and to give emergency primary surgical care on the field, as well as to remove the wounded from the sphere of fighting. His ambulant technique became possible with the development, under Napoléon's genius, of improved artillery strategies, unfettered cavalry for greater reconnaissance and maneuvering, and open-formation skirmishes spread over an extended front. Clearly, the earlier tactics of volley firing of troops standing shoulder-to-shoulder on open ground within two hundred yards of the enemy, followed by bayonet charge, made first aid and evacuation of the wounded during battle an almost impossible task.

With the consent of General Custine, Larrey procured several two- and four-wheeled light wagons, organizing them into the "flying ambulance" (*ambulance volante*), which he directed to move across the battlefield. These vehicles carried medical officers and their assistants and moved right into the front line, maintaining contact with the troops during the engagement. The wounded were brought directly to the surgeons by comrades or waited for the ambulance wagon to arrive where they had fallen. Once there, the wounded received immediate medical attention, with the surgeons performing amputations and extracting bullets. After the wounds were dressed, the injured were placed in the ambulance wagon and carried quickly to a nearby field hospital (*chirurgicie de bataille*). The inspiration for the flying hospital derived from several sources, including John Randby in England and the experiences of the French, English, Dutch, Hanoverian, and Austrian armies at Fontenoy (1745), where regimental surgeons had treated soldiers on the line and had then collected them at stations for transfer to hospitals.[18]

Larrey did not fully perfect his ambulance units until the Italian campaign of 1796, when he organized his system of *ambulance volantes*, with one unit for every ten thousand men. In total, each ambulance unit consisted of 340 men constituted into three divisions under the direction of a chief surgeon. To support a division, Larrey provided eight two-wheeled, two-horse wagons for use in flat country, and four four-wheeled, four-horse wagons intended for more hilly terrain to carry the wounded. Larrey's special wagon, distinct from the usual supply wagon, consisted of an oblong box suspended from springs, with doors at the front and rear, sliding shutters on the sides, and two padded litters on casters. The two-wheeled wagon (plate 1) carried two patients lying full length, while the four-wheeled wagon accommodated four wounded, although they had to lie with their legs bent. Larrey supported his special wagons with four storage wagons and one hundred support personnel, of whom fourteen were surgeons. After receiving official recognition for his successes, Larrey organized ambulance support for the Imperial Guard, including flying ambulances for Napoléon's Egyptian campaign of 1799.[19]

Like Ambroise Paré before him, Larrey recognized the benefits of immediate amputation while the wounded soldier was in shock and his limbs numb from pain. In his preface to *Memoir on Amputation*, Larrey noted that "the first four hours are an isolated period of calm which nature is able to maintain, and advantage should be taken of this to administer the appropriate remedy, as in any other dangerous malady." Under these circumstances, amputation was a relatively painless operation, although when the shock passed, control of hemorrhage often proved difficult.[20] Larrey found that amputations carried out a week or ten days after the injury resulted in a mortality rate of 90 percent or more, while those performed immediately following the injury reduced mortality to 25 percent or less.[21]

Another French surgeon, Pierre François Percy (1754–1825), serving under General Jean-Victor Moreau (1763–1813), also endeavored to improve medical support for the wounded on the battlefield. Distressed by unnecessary deaths due to undisciplined hospital attendants and disorganized transport, Percy organized a corps of surgeons for each division and designed a mobile hospital called a *Wurtz* (named for the Austrian wagon works but known popularly as "Percy's Wurst" because of its resemblance to a sausage) that, modeled on light artillery wagons, could move close to the battle and provide initial surgical support. Each wagon, drawn by six horses, carried hand stretchers, instruments, emergency supplies for twelve hundred wounded, eight surgeons, and a complement of 120 orderlies. Because it was too heavy and cumbersome for the battlefield, the surgical wagon remained in a safe area near the line, where it provided aid to those able to walk or who were carried by stretcher (plate 2).[22] The Percy surgical wagon became an initial hospital station for those unable to reach the larger hospital train several miles behind the line. The wagon demonstrated the value of medical assistance for soldiers who might otherwise have died from exposure or from their wounds, providing essential support until other arrangements could be made. Nevertheless, Percy's approach left those immobilized by their wounds on the field rather than removing them to safer ground.[23]

During Moreau's campaign in Spain in 1808, Percy resolved this problem by organizing a trained ambulance stretcher-bearer corps (*brancardiers*) to gather wounded during a battle and carry them to a surgical support station. Each bearer's lance became a litter pole, and the bearer's sash, one-half of the litter (plates 3, 4) when laced lengthwise. Any two *brancardiers* could thus combine their equipment to create a *brancard*, or litter. The army assigned thirty-two litter bearers to each company of hospital attendants; their responsibility was to carry wounded to organized dressing stations just behind the front lines. In the Decree of 1813, the French army formally recognized the *brancardier* system; it became the embryo of the later regimental bearer company. Anticipating the Geneva Convention of 1864, Percy also urged the neutralization of medical personnel and stores, including the ambulances and hospitals.[24]

According to Venant A. L. Legouest, in *Traité de chirurgie d'armée* (1863), the ideas of both Larrey and Percy, which were endorsed by Napoléon, laid the groundwork for the subsequent ambulance support systems adopted by most European armies. Notwithstanding Legouest's remarks, however, the endorsement by Napoléon extended only to Larrey and Percy and not to their plans for a permanent surgical corps for the entire French army. The emperor's distrust of doctors, combined with his belief that medical officers should not be an integral part of the army, prevented the full establishment of flying-hospital attachments. Moreover, other nations seemed not to notice or respond to Larrey's ideas, except perhaps in theory. Change came slowly, as the British and Russians could attest in the Crimea some fifty years later.[25]

By mid century, almost every European army employed some combination of stretcher-bearers and ambulance wagons. The Prussian army, for example, attached "bearer companies" to each army corps to aid the wounded and to assist in their removal from the battle lines. Each bearer company consisted of 202 noncommissioned officers and men, with forty-five hand litters, and twelve pairs of crutches. They were attached to the flying detachments of the light hospitals and assigned in each division within the corps. The flying detachment provided first aid to the wounded on the field of battle; the army restricted this aid to bandages, tourniquets, and other operations essential to preserving life. The flying detachment prevented soldiers from leaving ranks to carry their wounded comrades to safer positions in the rear, a situation that all too frequently became an excuse to avoid battle. The detachment also protected the wounded from thieves and marauders.[26]

A second line of support came in a sheltered position near the engagement, where five medical officers, an apothecary, and ten attendants received the wounded. Four ambulance wagons for severely wounded, a medicine and bandage wagon, and a reserve wagon supported this section. Finally, a third support group provided medical attention further in the rear of the battle zone; it was from this latter area, usually a village or farm, that the wounded were transported to fixed hospitals. This organizational scheme, originating out of the experiences of the French army, endured with minor changes into the First World War.[27]

THE CRIMEAN WAR

With Britain and France suspicious of Russian ambitions to secure an outlet from the landlocked Black Sea, Russia's efforts to liberate the Balkan peoples and occupy Constantinople resulted in a collective effort by the European powers to preserve the integrity of the Ottoman state. The resulting Crimean War lasted from September 14, 1854, to July 12, 1856, and concentrated principally on the siege of Sebastopol. Forces in the Crimea numbered: French, 309,268 (including 550 medical officers); English, 97,864 (448 medical officers); Russians, 324,478 (1,608 army surgeons); Sardinians, 21,000 (88 surgeons); and Turks, 35,000 (no reported medical personnel).[28]

The French army entered the Crimea prepared to wage war, with a complete ambulance system of army hospitals, including the flying and ordinary. To each division of infantry was attached an ambulance consisting of five line officers, six surgeons, three apothecaries, twenty male nurses, and an instrument maker and assistant. At the time of battle, the division ambulance divided into a *flying ambulance* (a light cart with one officer, two surgeons, and two *infirmiers*), which posted itself near the firing line to provide first aid and to evacuate the wounded. In addition, there was the *ordinary ambulance* (one officer, five surgeons, and twelve nurses) consisting of five carriages and more extensive medical matériel for fourteen hundred dressings. Both the flying and ordinary hospitals kept pace with the division's movements. At the beginning of the war, only forty hospital surgeons supported the ambulance and hospital service. By 1855, the number had increased to eighty-six.[29]

In contrast, the British were ill prepared to meet the needs of the wounded in the Crimea, and their medical evacuation system, such as it was, broke down with predictable regularity. Each British regiment had one surgeon and three assistant surgeons; a pack animal loaded with instruments, bandages, and medicines; and ten litters to support their medical needs. The army's ambulance wagons (two-wheeled carts drawn by two horses and four-wheelers drawn by six mules designed by Andrew Smith, director general of the Army and Ordnance Medical Department) did not disembark with the twenty-eight thousand troops at Varna, Bulgaria, in the summer of 1854. When they finally did arrive, there were no instructions for their assembly; as a result, the British moved into the Crimea without this essential support. In their place, raiding parties scoured the countryside and collected two dozen two-wheeled country carts to be used for medical support and evacuation. Complicating matters even more, Smith received inaccurate information on the size of the force required for the expedition, where the army would be fighting, and how long the fighting would last. Moreover, his warnings regarding climate, water supply, and local diseases went unheeded. From his offices at 13 St. James' Place, Smith and his meager staff of two assistant medical officers and four clerks set about to address the challenges of war in the absence of a medical plan. As Neil Cantlie explained, in *A History of the Army Medical Department* (1974), the "war was a glorious adventure and the glamour was not to be tarnished by a doctor's fads."[30]

The British army, which in previous wars had relied on drummers and bandsmen to serve as litter bearers, was unprepared for the large numbers of sick and wounded. Indeed, the Royal Expeditionary Force went to the Crimea with astonishing nonchalance. Smith's desire to create a hospital corps of six hundred men to serve as orderlies and ambulance drivers was accepted in principle by the secretary of state at war, but differences immediately arose over the source of men for the corps. The director general's request for volunteers from soldiers serving in India was abandoned for lack of response.[31] Thus, when England entered the war, it relied instead on civilians; but civilians lacked the discipline and habits of military life. To make matters worse, the military turned a deaf ear to Smith's proposal to hire eight hundred Armenians recruited in Turkey and placed under military control for ambulance duty. Eventually the Hospital Conveyance Corps, consisting of 370 pensioners, 20 four-wheeled wagons, 20 two-wheeled carts, and 9 Flanders store wagons, organized independently of the War Office to serve the sick and wounded. Intended for allocation to the divisions, the four-wheeled wagons proved too heavy and cumbersome for the small Bulgarian horses, and the two-wheeled ambulance wagons tipped over on bad roads and, in general, caused great discomfort to the sick and wounded. Arriving in Varna in

July during the height of the cholera epidemic, 104 of the corpsmen fell victim to the disease and consequently provided little support to the British expeditionary forces. Of the remaining corpsmen, many became drunken nuisances who proved little assistance in attending to the sick and wounded.[32]

Casualties soon cluttered the wharves and were packed into ships that lacked proper facilities, hospital support staff, or even kitchens. Hospital vessels, such as the *Cambria*, *Andes*, *John Masterson*, and *Kangaroo*, evacuated the sick and wounded from Varna to Scutari. Inadequate for the numbers, these and other transport vessels became little more than death ships crammed beyond reasonable capacity and lacking in surgeons and orderlies.[33]

While the French situated their hospitals on the European side of the Dardanelles, the British, with the exception of a naval hospital at Therapia, located theirs at Scutari, on the Asiatic side across the water from Constantinople. Like the medical transport vessels, the Scutari hospitals were little more than "dead houses," as one young Edinburgh doctor described them. Moreover, many of the paid nurses proved "unskilled, disorderly, and a number were too fond of the bottle."[34] At the Koulali Hospital, one of every four patients died of fever, dysentery, or infection, in part because the hospital had originally served as a Turkish cavalry barracks early in the war and had never been properly cleaned. The medical officers and their staffs were attacked by the various parasites that came in with the men from the front. Most soldiers suffered from scurvy, and many died from hemorrhages. After serving in the Crimean War for fourteen months, a Russian surgeon, Nikolai I. Pirogoff (1810–81), described the war as "an epidemic of trauma."[35]

Lack of proper clothing and rations and rampant cholera and dysentery created situations of unmanageable proportions. Doctors issued cholera belts, curtailed parades, ordered encampments to change frequently, and prohibited wine and the eating of unripe fruit. No one suggested simply boiling water, and to make matters worse, most regiments left behind their six-month medicine chests, relying instead on the packhorse and panniers with their one-week's supply of drugs.

Accompanying the Royal Expeditionary Force were 150 regular doctors who held diplomas from the royal colleges and who relied upon bloodletting, purgatives, and diaphoretics as the time-tested remedies for hospital gangrene, erysipelas, pyemia, and other inflammatory diseases. The department issued medical officers a copy of George J. Guthrie's *Commentaries on Surgery*, which dated back to the Peninsular War (1808–14) but which contained the only practical instruction on the problems of war surgery. In the absence of germ theory, antisepsis and the etiology of cholera remained unknowns, and opinions continued to differ over the advantages of immediate amputation on the field or later amputation in the hospital. In general, physicians in the Crimea agreed with Larrey (and Paré before him) on the benefits of immediate amputation. The only problem was knowing which cases demanded it and whether to operate when the wounded soldier was in shock. Little guidance existed on methods for anesthesia in surgery; some doctors, for example, preferred to carry out amputations with "the smart of the knife" rather than with chloroform. Despite a vocal minority of surgeons, chloroform became the most popular form of anesthetic.[36]

Soon after arriving, the British and French met the Russians on the heights of Alma on September 20, 1854; the British casualties numbered two thousand killed and wounded. While the English home front took pride in the crossing of the Alma River and the storming of the heights above, there was a public outcry when correspondent William Howard Russell reported on the official incompetence and the sufferings of the sick and wounded. Until Russell's dispatch in the *Times* on October 9, 1854, the English public had no reason to suspect that the war was going poorly for the soldiers. His dispatches, however, caused enough political pressure to force Sir Sidney Herbert, secretary of state at war, to ask Florence Nightingale to organize a group of trained female nurses for duty in the Crimea. Appointed superintendent of the Female Nursing Establishment of the English General Hospital in Turkey, she set out with thirty-eight other women whom she had selected, arriving on November 4, ten days after the battle of Balaclava.

The battle of Balaclava on October 25, 1854, with its famous "Charge of the Light Brigade," followed by the battle of Inkerman on November 5, created continued crises in medical support and evacuation. Shortages of doctors, dressings, chloroform, splints, and transport delayed emergency aid to the wounded and timely evacuation to the hospitals at Scutari. By December, more than a third of the British forces had died or were suffering from malaria, dysentery, typhoid fever, frostbite, cholera, or other diseases. Miss Nightingale reported a 43-percent mortality rate among patients admitted to the hospitals. As of July 12, 1856, when the last soldier left the Crimea, 16,297 of the 21,000 British deaths resulted from disease, not from battle injuries. Over the course of the war, however, the death rate declined from 293 per 1,000 soldiers in September, 1854, to 25 per 1,000 following the public outcry. Clearly, the influence of Florence Nightingale and the subsequent establishment of stricter sanitary controls resulted in a more effective medical support system for the troops.[37]

Overall, the war found the Army and Ordnance Medical Department unprepared for duties in the Crimea, administratively undertrained in the needs of active service, deficient in the most basic medical supplies, and lacking in ambulance transport and in essential hospital staffing. The high incidence of death and morbidity from diarrhea, dysentery, cholera, fever, scurvy, tetanus, amputation, frostbite, and gangrene affected morale both in the army and at the home front. Nevertheless, the war was not without some redeeming value. Amputation techniques improved; and the prefabricated wooden hospitals at Renkioi, designed on the pavilion system and built by Isambard Brunel, were an innovation in maintaining essential accommodations for the sick and wounded. Equally important, Florence Nightingale and her nurses won grudging respect from physicians and from the military, becoming an important factor in the medical support system and a force in the humanitarian efforts soon to capture the attention of the international community.[38]

AMERICA'S EARLY WARS

During the early days of the American Revolution, the Massachusetts regimental surgeons assumed responsibility for the sick and wounded, with their medical equipment and supplies provided by the Committee of Safety and the Committee of Supplies. This situation changed with the appointment of George Washington to command the Continental army and the spread of fighting into the colonies further south. However, the Continental army's Hospital Department (established in July 1775) did little to resolve the confusion that existed with respect to the supply of necessary medicines, the proper chain of command (including the role of the Congress), and the failure to explain the relationship between the department and the existing regimental system. To head the Hospital Department, the Continental Congress chose Dr. Benjamin Church, who had been active in the development and operation of the hospital system established for the Massachusetts military units. His appointment, however, proved short-lived due to opposition from regimental surgeons and, to everyone's embarrassment, his treasonous sharing of vital military information with the British. Dr. John Morgan succeeded Church and proceeded to organize the Hospital Department until his dismissal from the army in 1777, when George Washington's choice, Dr. William Shippen, was appointed to succeed him. Reflecting the spirited regionalism of the Congress and its distrust of anything hinting of centralization, the army's medical establishment faced numerous intrigues and opposition from those who preferred a decentralized system of regimental hospitals and medical care.[39]

Throughout the revolutionary war, the army's Hospital Department remained a hotbed of internecine feuds (with villains both inside and outside the department) and the source of appalling misdirection. The confusion, however, stemmed as much from the Continental Congress as it did from its own mismanagement. At its best, the department directed efforts toward providing competent physicians and surgeons, sufficient medical supplies, and capable nurses. However, there was no assurance from military policies and procedures that what the department directed had much impact at the field or regimental hospitals located in the rear of the army. And, as in England, the medical support system remained in the rear during the fighting and attended only those able to reach there. Those unable to leave the field (with or without the aid of comrades) waited for the battle to end before being attended by a regimental surgeon's mate or by the surgeon himself. Later, they were brought by carts, improvised litters, wagons, or horseback to flying hospitals in the rear, which consisted of tents containing six beds and an operating table and managed by the Continental military establishment. Further behind the line, the Continental army managed general hospitals located in churches, private homes, and barns. Transportation of the wounded was accomplished with the help of servants, bandsmen, local inhabitants, volunteers, and impressed workers who, using any available means (wheelbarrows, oxteams, and army supply wagons), carried out this errand of mercy.[40]

In the decades after the war, medical support for the army remained confused and unequal to the tasks before it. Alternating periods of active hostility and demobilization had a further demoralizing effect on those few visionaries who saw the need for a long-range plan of medical care for the nation's soldiers but who were unable to make a convincing argument. Not until 1818 did Congress establish a permanent Hospital Department with some semblance of long-term objectives. By then, even the most critical opponents had at last recognized the lessons so painfully learned from costly indifference and the lack of preparedness.[41]

By the time of the Mexican War (1846–48), the United States was no more prepared medically to support its troops than the British were in the Crimea; the army had no vehicles designed specifically to serve as army ambulances before 1859. Instead, it relied on 180 mule-drawn wagons available in the spring of 1847. Ignorance of hygiene resulted in 10,951 deaths from disease, while only 1,549 died of wounds. This meant a disease rate of 110 per 1,000, compared with 65 per 1,000 in the Civil War and 16 per 1,000 in the First World War.[42]

During the Crimean War, Secretary of War Jefferson Davis sent a military commission of Majors Richard Delafield (1798–1873) and

Alfred Mordecai (1804–87) and Captain George B. McClellan (1826–85) to visit the war theater and to report on any new systems of warfare. Davis also directed them to observe "the kind of ambulances or other means used for transporting the sick and wounded." Delafield's subsequent account of the armies in the Crimea described the ambulance systems adopted by the French, English, Russian, and other European armies.[43] In his *Report to the Senate* in June 1860, Delafield explained the use of ambulance transport in the war, especially during the siege of Sebastopol. He praised the work of Florence Nightingale and described the various carriages employed by the British and Russian armies and the wrought-iron chairs or litters that hung like packsaddles on mules. He also examined the English hospital train of twenty carts, which served twelve regiments and consisted of a sergeant major, four other noncommissioned officers, a staff surgeon, and sixty-nine drivers and attendants. These arrangements for moving the wounded from the battlefield to camp and field hospitals, and finally to general hospitals near Constantinople, would serve as models during the Civil War.[44]

THE AMERICAN CIVIL WAR

When the War of the Rebellion broke out in April 1861 following General Pierre Beauregard's bombardment of Fort Sumter, Americans—both North and South—were unprepared to wage war on such a large scale. Except during the Mexican War, the United States had never maintained an army of more than twenty-five thousand men. For that reason, few had ever considered the need for medical care of forces larger than a few regiments. The military system itself reflected the habits and traditions of a small nation, whose combatants were ill equipped to understand the consequences of a civil rebellion, much less a war that would end in unconditional surrender.

In December 1861, two hundred regiments, or 176,042 men, assembled on the Potomac River; of that number, 7.3 percent, or 12,841, required immediate hospital support—not from battle wounds but from diarrhea, dysentery, typhus, measles, smallpox, fever, and other diseases aggravated by inadequate clothing, bad water, and poor food. At the outbreak of the war, the nation had no army general hospital, and the Medical Corps of the U.S. Army amounted to a mere thirty surgeons and eighty-three assistant surgeons. Of that number, three surgeons and twenty-one assistant surgeons resigned to join the Confederacy. The army dismissed an additional three assistant surgeons for disloyalty. And, typical of regional loyalty, surgeons attached to volunteer units often refused to accept wounded who were not of their own outfit or state.

Within twenty-eight months of the beginning of the war, twelve hundred volunteer surgeons were working with the armies in the field. By November 1862, the North had 150 general hospitals attending 60,500 sick and wounded.[45] By 1864, 192 general and special Union army hospitals were operational. The largest were Harewood (2,000 beds) and Lincoln (2,575) in Washington, D.C.; Mower (3,100) and Satterlee (3,519) in Philadelphia; Jefferson (2,399) in Indiana; and the U.S. General Hospital (3,497) near Fortress Monroe in Virginia.[46]

Fearing that American soldiers might face sanitary debacles, such as those the soldiers of the Crimea had endured, humanitarian organizations, including the Women's Central Association of Relief, Bellevue Hospital, and other public and private institutions, insisted upon a formalized agency to support the medical needs of the combatants. Not until June 13, 1861, however, did Abraham Lincoln approve the establishment of the United States Sanitary Commission, more to assuage public pressure than because of a genuine belief in its efficacy. Organized in New York City by Reverend Henry W. Bellows (1814–82), a Unitarian minister who served as its honorary first president, the Sanitary Commission was modeled after the British support groups in the Crimea and became known derogatively as "Lincoln's fifth wheel," meaning that it was as useful as a "fifth wheel to a coach." Opposition came from the Medical Department itself, which claimed that the commission had exaggerated problems and issues, and from Edwin M. Stanton, Lincoln's second secretary of war. Key supporters of the commission included Alexander D. Bache; Professor Jeffries Wyman, M.D.; Wolcott Gibbs, M.D.; Samuel G. Howe, M.D.; and W. H. Van Buren, M.D.[47]

Sanitary Commission General Secretary Frederick Law Olmstead (1822–1903) supervised its day-to-day operation and organized "sanitary fairs" in the major cities of the North to support its work. Providing advice, as well as material aid, to the Medical Department (which Olmstead found particularly inept) and exposing negligence and incompetence wherever found, commission workers forced the government and the military to accept greater responsibility for the sick and wounded. The commission became one of the "great moral and physical forces" of the Civil War, urging not only the revitalization of the Medical Department but recommending the appointment of thirty-three-year-old physician William A. Hammond (1828–1900) as surgeon general in place of the elderly Clement A. Finley. Commission activities included purchasing medical supplies and equipment, providing nurses, caring for refugees, urging more exacting physical examinations of recruits, advocating the inspection of camps and hospitals, focusing attention on sanitation and on disease prevention, collecting donations, lobbying for reorganization of the Medical Department, urging the transfer of transportation service for the sick and wounded from the Quartermaster's Department to the Medical Department, and assisting in the establishment of a permanent ambulance service. In addition, the commission offered assistance to the sick and wounded (including war prisoners), urged the creation of a nursing corps, provided ambulances and medical supplies to armies in the field, and helped families and relatives locate wounded soldiers. Branches of the commission existed in Boston, Cincinnati, Chicago, and six other cities.[48]

St. Louis became the headquarters of the military's Department of the West, and during the summer of 1861, following the battles of Boonville, Dug Spring, Carthage, and Wilson's Creek, wounded were transported to the city in ambulances, army wagons, and railroad cars. There, their plight aroused the sympathies of benevolent citizens. Dorothea Dix, who was in St. Louis at the time, called upon Major General John C. Frémont; his wife, Jessie; and "other persons of humane and patriotic motives and sentiments [who] were personally known to General Frémont," to establish a Sanitary Commission "to be subordinate to and act in aid of the Medical Department." At the suggestion of Unitarian minister William Greenleaf Eliot, businessmen James Erwin Yeatman and C. S. Greeley; J. B. Johnson, M.D.; George Partridge; and a number of other St. Louis doctors, businessmen, and philanthropists, General Frémont recognized the Western Sanitary Commission to aid soldiers in Missouri. Organized separately from its eastern cousin to support the armies, the navy, and the hospitals west of the Mississippi, the western commission was soon to rival the national commission.[49]

Viewed with suspicion by the Medical Department and by the army, the Western Sanitary Commission was initially excluded from supporting the regular army and could operate only with the navy, providing needed stores on the Mississippi River. Eventually, the western commission directed relief operations to the armies west of the Mississippi, fitting out hospital steamers and transporting supplies to gunboats on the river; it maintained hospital stores, established soldiers' homes, assigned women nurses, and cared for refugees, including some forty thousand blacks. The commission provided assistance and protection for blacks until these duties were taken over by the National Freedmen's Relief Association in New York City, the Northwestern Freedmen's Relief Commission in Chicago, and similar organizations in Cincinnati, Indianapolis, and elsewhere.[50]

In the fall of 1862, the western commission also attempted to organize a flying hospital to accompany the army in the field to attend to the needs of the wounded. To accomplish this, commission personnel fitted out three ambulance wagons, which they supported with a corps of male nurses and wound dressers. Approved by Assistant Surgeon General Robert C. Wood, the first of the flying hospitals went to General Ulysses S. Grant's army at Corinth, Mississippi. Medical Director Horace R. Wirtz, however, refused to permit the hospital to proceed and scuttled the enterprise, deeming it unnecessary. He returned the mules and ambulances to the soldiers' homes at Columbus and Memphis and the supplies to hospitals at La Grange, Kentucky, and elsewhere.[51] Ironically, the same suspicion and jealousy that existed between the Medical Department and the commissions, existed as well among the U.S. Sanitary Commission, the Western Sanitary Commission, and the Christian Sanitary Commission. Protective of their respective autonomy and proud of their regional hegemony, they chose to go their separate ways in the conflict.[52]

AMBULANCE ORGANIZATION

Like most military establishments, the United States Army operated under the aegis of the *Regulations for the Army of the United States*, first issued by the War Office in 1808. The first mention of medical transportation occurred in the 1814 *Regulations* as one of the duties of regimental surgeons but referred only to those men permitted to ride in available baggage wagons and to the allocation of a two-horse wagon to each regimental hospital to carry medicines, blankets, and other hospital stores. Although the document defined the duties of medical officers, it ignored transportation for the wounded until the reorganization of the army in 1821, when the revised *Regulations* compiled by General Winfield Scott (1786–1866) gave the Army Medical Department certain discretion in this area and authorized the medical director to establish field or movable hospitals and, in concert with the quartermaster general, "cause a suitable number of light wagons and attendants to be attached to the several parts of the field hospital, each detachment under the conduct of an officer or agent of the Quartermaster's Department. When practicable, these attendants will be selected from the country people." An 1825 revision applied the term *ambulance* to the field or movable hospitals stationed behind the line of battle and, as in the 1821 revision, directed the Quartermaster's Department, after consultation with the medical director, to provide the wounded with light wagons and attendants hired on contract.[53]

In reflecting on this new theory of ambulance support, W. E. Horner, in the *American Cyclopedia of Practical Medicine and Surgery* for 1834, recommended that the ambulance was "to afford . . . the wounded a prompt and easy transportation from the ranks while in combat, to concentrate a body of medical men upon any particular point or points of an extended line of battle, and to transport along with them their instruments, medicines, and nurses." For soldiers, this ambulance service, or flying hospital, assured them that medical assistance was at hand and that slight wounds could be treated prior to their returning to battle.[54]

As part of the military train, the ambulance organization followed the movements of the division, subject to orders from headquarters. Ambulance service served as an auxiliary, its equipment distinct from the more formal-medical service of the regiments. The ambulance organization had many features of a hospital without the encumbrances of a permanent station. Its obligations to wounded soldiers lasted only a short time: attending the immediate needs of the wounded, transferring them to a stationary hospital, and leaving again to follow the combat. For that reason, medical officers omitted every nonessential piece of equipment that might delay or otherwise burden the ambulance wagon and its support staff.[55]

Under battle conditions, medical officers and their support moved to the rear of the action "at a sufficient distance from the range of cannon-shot." There, they set up tents near adjoining settlements or houses to administer to the wounded. While one portion of the corps remained at this temporary station to accept the wounded, the rest moved with their carriages as near the action as possible. At the carriages, essential treatment consisted of stopping hemorrhages and maintaining the wounded until they either returned to their regiments or moved to the nearest stationary hospital. Surgeons with battle experience did not recommend amputations or excisions at the first bandaging station because doing so meant others would go without aid.[56]

Assuming fifteen hundred men wounded in three separate engagements out of a body of six or seven thousand troops, Horner calculated that the minimum ambulance organization required the services of a chief surgeon, two junior surgeons, six assistant surgeons, a quartermaster, an experienced cutler to maintain instruments, a steward, and fifty nurses. Armies also would hire women to wash, cook, and provide additional nursing care for the wounded. Horner estimated that two carriages could convey needed instruments and hospital stores. These carriages consisted of a long box that was cushioned on the ridge for seating and was divided into two rows of compartments for instruments, surgical dressings, splints, medicines, camphorated spirits, and brandy. Four carriages transported the sick and wounded. Attendants laid the worst cases on thick mattresses spread on the floor, while less serious cases sat on seats at each side. These four carriages traveled across the field of battle, picking up soldiers as they went. Hand litters provided additional support.[57]

Despite the comprehensiveness of Horner's plan, subsequent revisions of the *Regulations* in 1834, 1835, and 1841 provided only narrow interpretations for assistance to the sick and wounded. "For the accommodation of the sick and disabled a wagon will be attached to the rear guard when necessary and practicable, and a surgeon will attend and give assistance and to see that no improper persons are suffered to avail themselves of the accommodation." With the sudden outbreak of war between the United States and Mexico, the 1847 *Regulations* were issued without substantive revision of its medical system for field service. Accordingly, the Medical Department remained dependent for transportation on the Quartermaster's Department. Notwithstanding this impediment, an ad hoc system evolved during the Mexican War giving substantial freedom to the Medical Department. Some of these elements were embodied in the 1857 revision. Still, the quartermaster made "all necessary arrangements for the transportation of the wounded."[58]

The Civil War rudely awakened the American people to the need for an effective ambulance system. Although early efforts to provide ambulance support had occurred in the War of 1812 and in the campaigns in Florida and Mexico, the first organized American ambulance system dated to the establishment of the U.S. Army Medical Board on October 18, 1859. This board, consisting of Assistant Surgeon Richard H. Coolidge, Surgeons Clement A. Finley, Richard S. Satterlee, John M. Cuyler, and Charles S. Tripler, reviewed various ambulance models, adopting the four-wheeled Tripler and the two-wheeled Finley and Coolidge models for test trials at several posts in the western service. When the Civil War began, no organized ambulance service existed between the first-aid station at the front and the base hospitals in the rear. In keeping with the 1857 *Regulations*, two- and four-wheeled vehicles remained under the control of the Quartermaster's Department, which assigned them as needed—and only temporarily—to medical duties. Not until March 1864 would Congress approve the creation of a uniform ambulance system.[59]

The *Regulations* of 1861 continued the bifurcated responsibility between the Medical Department and the Quartermaster's Department, requiring that the quartermaster arrange all transportation of the wounded, establish ambulance depots and hospitals in the rear, and instruct those responsible for removing the wounded. Lacking a system for training and lacking as well any medical inspectors, the Medical Department limped along in the early days of the war, learning from its experiences—tragic as many of them were—before demonstrating the ability to accommodate the medical needs of the wounded.[60]

"At the outbreak of the Civil War," wrote Captain Louis C. Duncan, author of *The Medical Department of the United States Army in the Civil War* (1985), "there was in the United States Army neither plan, personnel, nor equipment for collecting the wounded from the battlefield, caring for them in [a] hospital, or transporting them to the rear." No ambulance corps existed despite Larrey's trailblazing efforts in Napoléon's Grand Army. At best, the typical regiment of six or seven hundred men carried into battle a half-dozen two-horse Finley or Coolidge ambulance wagons and two or three tents, which held no more than eight men each; hospital supplies and litters hardly existed, and army regulations permitted only bandsmen to use the equipment.[61] Medical service centered on the needs of the regiment, with no plan for evacuation beyond this unit. Thus, the army thought in terms of regimental ambulances, hospitals, supplies, and personnel. Exemplifying this narrow thinking, General Irvin McDowell authorized only fifty ambulance wagons for his entire army of thirty-five thousand.[62]

In 1861, Surgeon T. H. Squire of the Eighty-ninth New York Volunteers noted that any plan to care for battle-wounded required an understanding of the organization and disposition of the army during military engagements. Using a tree as illustrative of an army corps, Squire compared the root with headquarters, the main branches with the three divisions of the corps, subdivisions of the three branches for the nine brigades, smaller limbs representing the thirty-six regiments, and twigs representing the 360 companies. Armies of any large size would consist of several of these military trees planted side by side and forming a battle line that stretched across the war theater.[63]

Reflecting the orderliness of this organization, the battle-wounded—those able to help themselves from the field and those requiring assistance—followed very specific procedures. Soldiers able to travel without assistance reported to the nearest officer for permission to leave the line. They then reported to the regimental hospital, where a steward registered their names. A medical officer examined and dressed their wounds before directing them to proceed with a written pass to the divisional hospital. There, they again registered, had their wounds redressed if necessary, and then moved to the corps hospital for treatment or to a general hospital beyond the theater of military operation.[64]

Physicians performed all surgical operations at the division hospital, which the army established close to the line of battle but distant enough to be safe from cannon- and rifleshot. In Squire's opinion, the most sensible organizational design for the division hospital was a wheel (plate 5), with the chief surgeon at the center; the hospital stewards, medicines, and dressings occupying the innermost zone; the operating surgeons and their tables the second zone; the ambulances the third; the wards for the wounded the fourth; the transportation wagons the fifth zone; the kitchens and the commissary stores the sixth; and the hospital guards the final zone.

Upon their initial arrival at the division hospital, the wounded rested on straw, hay, corn husks, paper, feathers, dried seaweed, bran, leaves, or sawdust strewn around the ground for their comfort. Sawdust made from pine proved to be an especially useful aseptic base for mattresses and pillows. The amputating tables were either part of the regular apparatus of the hospital or "extemporaneously constructed of materials obtained from neighboring houses." For splints, pads, or cushions, the battlefield offered a variety of articles from which to improvise.[65]

Properly organized, argued Squire, the division hospital became an efficient medical center. Ambulances entered the inner zone, where soldiers were classified according to the urgency of their wounds, the severe cases being cared for immediately and other cases arranged on the basis of need. Wounded remained at the division hospital no longer than was necessary to apply dressings, administer medicines, and provide food. Personnel then transported the wounded by railroad, hospital ship, wagon, or carriage to the corps hospital for further treatment.

As carefully planned as Squire's organizational scheme appeared, it was far from the reality experienced by most soldiers during the Civil War. Instead, surgeons performed field surgery with unclean knives, sponges, and bullet probes; used waxed harness maker's silk or horsehair for ligatures; and explored with surgically unclean hands. Needless to say, patients contracted septicemia pyemia, erysipelas, hospital gangrene, and even tetanus. Most of the tetanus occurred at Antietam, Stones River, and Fredericksburg, where stables were used as field hospitals. Equally troublesome was the medical field service, which was responsible for removing the wounded from the battlefield and transporting them to dressing stations. As in earlier wars in America and Europe, the military detailed regimental musicians and convalescents to serve as stretcher-bearers, while hired civilians drove horse-drawn conveyances of various types.[66]

To complicate matters further, improvements in military arms and munitions, most notably rifling and the conoidal bullet with percussion cap and fixed ammunition, brought increased effective range to the battlefield and forced tactics—and medical evacuation procedures—to adjust accordingly. The zones of enemy fire increased in depth as the precision of the newer rifles caused thinning and lengthening of lines. Wounded were scattered over larger areas than before, requiring sanitary corpsmen to spread their medical support system across a broader front. This spread meant situating several surgeons and a hospital with each regiment, establishing a mobile hospital under canvas with each division, and organizing numerous fixed hospitals at military bases and elsewhere beyond the war theater. This undertaking proved to be both cumbersome and impractical, often interfering with the tactical mobility of the army. Between the firing line and the division hospitals, and from the division hospitals to the base hospitals, little mobile sanitary organization existed.[67]

In May 1861, Dr. J. O. Bronson of New York urged General Winfield Scott to organize aides, nurses, and sufficient men to attend ambulances and litters. In September 1861, Dr. H. H. Smith, the surgeon general of Pennsylvania, made a similar plea, followed the next spring by Charles Pfirsching, whose proposal resembled Percy's stretcher-bearer corps (*brancardiers*) already in place in Europe.

> To every division of the army a company shall be attached which will follow it immediately into action on the day of battle for the purpose of taking up all its wounded and carrying them back to the ambulances, or to the points where the regimental surgeons have taken position. Each man of this company should be armed and equipped in the following manner: Two navy revolvers, carried in the cartridge-box belt; a hatchet, carried on the left side of the cartridge-box belt; a cartridge-box on a leather belt; a knapsack half filled with his own things, while the other half is appropriated to a stock of bandages, linen, lint, etc., as they may be necessary for a bandage to prevent the death of the wounded before he obtains the assistance of the surgeon. Besides some prepared sticking plasters, etc., and some bottles with stimulating essences to recall the spirits of the wounded, or to enable him to bear the pains of his wound and of the transportation, a large canteen with water, to which some vinegar or pure brandy may be added for the use of the wounded; a thin tumbler with it; a small canteen for the man's own use; a small box on the cartridge-box belt, with lint, bandages, a small bottle of vinegar for immediate use, so that he has not to take off the knapsack; the half of a litter of my own invention. Two men of this company always keep together, and by means of their two halves they form a litter on which they carry the wounded from the battlefield to the ambulances, or to the places where the regimental surgeons have established themselves.[68]

Ironically, Surgeon Charles S. Tripler's response to Pfirsching noted that, however sound the scheme appeared on paper, there was nothing new in the plan, and, moreover, it was too late to establish such a complicated support organization. Instead, Tripler assigned ten soldiers and bandsmen to ambulance service.[69]

Recognizing the meagerness of the medical support in the early days of the war, Surgeon Henry S. Hewit, who served with General Grant's army at Fort Donelson in February 1862, chose to group his regimental hospitals at one location, close to the rear, and supplemented this support with additional shelter in farmhouses and other buildings. However, Hewit provided no arrangements for further evacuation. In contrast, Surgeon Thomas A. McParlin, with General John Pope's army in August 1862, organized a clearing hospital directly behind the corps from which his soldiers were evacuated by rail to hospitals in the rear. Although conceptually sound, the plan failed for lack of sufficient ambulance support service and for the inaccessibility of the clearing hospital to base hospitals. As a result, soldiers collected at the clearing hospital remained a week or more before being evacuated.[70]

Dr. Henry I. Bowditch (1809–92) raised public alarm when, during a visit to Washington, D.C., in September 1862, he characterized the existing ambulance system as an atrocity and demanded a more humane solution. At the suggestion of Surgeon General William A. Hammond, Bowditch joined a train of carriages hastily organized on September 5 to carry relief to the starving and wounded near Centreville, Virginia, following the second battle of Bull Run (August 29–30). As in the wars of previous centuries, the army had focused wholly upon the results of battle, giving little or no consideration to caring for the wounded. In fact, the army had made no hospital arrangements at all and had provided no plan for transporting the wounded.[71]

The ambulance train, which started with fifty carriages, was quickly reduced to forty-seven when three drivers refused to enter enemy lines, a desertion made easy because they were civilians and lacked military escort. Bowditch described the drivers as "men of the lowest character, evidently taken from the vilest purlieus of Washington, merely as common drivers, and for no other qualifications." His own driver's lack of skill caused Bowditch to assume control of a carriage in which he had begun as a passenger.[72] According to Bowditch's account, the wagon train lacked any semblance of discipline and, by the following morning, was strung out in almost total disregard for its mission. Once, the train stopped altogether as drivers ran into a nearby field to forage for apples and peaches. Here, under the flag of truce, wagon drivers trespassed on a planter's property to plunder. The ambulance train finally arrived at midday, finding soldiers "in a most piteous condition, lying everywhere, inside and outside of every building connected with a small farmhouse."

Once there, the drivers refused to attend the wounded, and only after much persuasion did they agree to carry water to aid in dressing wounds. On the return trip to Washington, Bowditch observed that several intoxicated drivers had actually fallen backwards from their seats onto the wounded.[73]

Although alarmist in tone and intent, Bowditch's findings were by no means atypical. The *New York Times* and *Medical Times* recounted similar stories. A physician who served at Manassas recalled that "the ambulance drivers behaved in the most disgraceful manner, refusing to assist in removing the wounded unless whiskey was furnished them. They also robbed the wounded of blankets provided for their comfort, and broke into the hospital stores and drank a portion of the liquor."[74]

As a result of his experiences near Centreville, Bowditch effectively utilized the prestige and reputation of the Massachusetts Medical Society to generate public sentiment in support of "a real ambulance corps." His efforts succeeded when, in October, Josiah Bartlett, president of the society, reported on the "gross abuses" of the ambulance service and urged the members of the society and the medical community in general to demand that the Medical Department of the United States Army be given "immediate supervision of the ambulance division, and, if possible, that a real ambulance corps should be established."[75]

HAMMOND AND LETTERMAN

Surgeon General Hammond, the principal catalyst for reform of the Medical Department of the Union army, inherited a department fossilized by incompetent leadership and an archaic organizational structure. With previous experience in the army and as a former professor of anatomy and physiology at the University of Maryland, he moved vigorously to introduce new ideas and new blood into the military's antiquated system. His immediate measures included a system for disease classification, accurate record keeping, and improved procurement. As early as 1862, Hammond recommended the creation of a permanent hospital and ambulance corps, the establishment of an army medical school and a permanent general hospital in Washington, and the independence of the Medical Department from the Quartermaster's Department.

Despite his achievements, Hammond's personality made him difficult, if not impossible, to work with. His lack of tact and his impulsive temper, combined with allegations of fraud and a series of controversial decisions, including the elimination of calomel and tartar emetic from the Standard Supply Table (a decision that caused him to be branded by regular physicians as an ally of medical sectarianism), brought his dismissal by

Stanton in November 1863. Believing he would be vindicated if judged fairly, Hammond sought immediate reinstatement or court-martial. He received the latter; and, on August 13, 1864, following a particularly vindictive trial, he was discharged in disgrace from the service. Hammond remained, however, a strong advocate of the Medical Department, insisting on greater efficiency and higher standards. Ultimately, and in spite of his arrogance, he was more than vindicated by his reforms, which proved effective in Europe and in the United States in the decades following the Civil War. Not until 1879 did Congress and President Rutherford B. Hayes annul the court's sentence.[76]

As surgeon general, Hammond had publicly argued for the establishment of an ambulance corps. "In no battle yet," he wrote, "have the wounded been properly looked after; men under pretence of carrying them off the field leave the ranks and seldom return to their proper duties. The adoption of this plan would do away with the necessity of taking men from the line of the army to perform the duties of nurses, cooks, and attendants, and thus return sixteen thousand men to duty in the ranks." Hammond's request went unanswered. Instead, hospital attendants (ten men to a regiment) and regimental bandsmen continued their duties as litter bearers and ambulance drivers.[77]

Although Hammond failed in his bid to establish a permanent hospital and ambulance corps, a situation that forced individual field commanders to resort to their own devices for handling the sick and wounded, he did convince General McClellan to appoint Jonathan Letterman (1824–72) in July 1862 as the medical director of the Army of the Potomac, succeeding Dr. Tripler, who had been medical director since August 12, 1861. A graduate of Jefferson Medical College who had spent twelve years in the Medical Department of the army, Letterman brought to the office a level of experience and enthusiasm that eventually transformed the medical service. In addition, his experiences at Harrison's Landing and his discussions with Hammond had given early indication of plans he formulated to improve the efficiency and responsiveness of the Medical Department.

On August 2, 1862, McClellan implemented General Orders No. 147, authorizing Letterman (with the support of Hammond) to organize an ambulance system within the Army of the Potomac. Letterman replaced the regimental medical service with a divisional service supported by a corps ambulance service. Under the direction of a captain, first lieutenants were charged with serving the division ambulances, second lieutenants with ambulances serving brigades, and sergeants with ambulances serving each regiment—all of whom were under the control of medical directors. The transportation allowance outlined in Letterman's plan provided for one transport cart; one four-horse and two two-horse ambulances for each regiment; one two-horse ambulance for each battery; and two two-horse ambulances for corps headquarters. Each ambulance carried two litters, with two men and a driver detailed from the line to operate the ambulance. Rather than use regimental musicians to act as litter bearers, Letterman preferred soldiers detailed and trained for the work. He also insisted that the ambulances in each division remain together to prevent line officers from using them for nonmedical purposes. Letterman thus removed from the Quartermaster Corps the responsibility for medical transportation and placed it under himself as medical director of the Army of the Potomac.[78]

Letterman also organized a field-hospital system for each division (rather than for each regiment), supported by a surgeon, two assistant surgeons, three medical officers to perform operations, and three additional officers to assist. In addition, he directed one assistant surgeon in each regiment to establish a first-aid station close to the battle line, with litter bearers as the conduit to the field hospitals.[79]

Due to the lack of ambulances and to the haste with which arrangements had been made, the advantages of this organization were only minimally witnessed at the battle of Antietam in September 1862. Although Antietam proved to be one of the bloodiest battles in American history, on a battle line six miles long, Letterman collected the wounded with three hundred ambulance wagons, one for each 175 men. The wagons moved to within a half mile of the battle line and waited for the wounded. With Union casualties of 12,410 and Confederate of 13,724, ambulance support units worked feverishly for two days to clear the wounded from the field to seventy-four improvised field hospitals in the vicinity. The ambulance corps then transferred the wounded from field hospitals to improvised clearing hospitals at Frederick, where the wounded were then evacuated to general hospitals in Baltimore, Washington, and Philadelphia. Even so, men wounded before noon on Wednesday remained unattended where they had fallen until Friday. Despite impediments, Letterman had demonstrated the unequivocal need for an ambulance system.[80]

Not until the battle of Fredericksburg (December 13, 1862) did Letterman fully test his medical evacuation system. By this time, too, the military had acquired medical supplies sufficient to equip its units prior to battle. General Ambrose E. Burnside, for example, provided nearly a thousand ambulances to support battle casualties. The fighting went on throughout the day; at nightfall, the ambulance corps began clearing the field of more than nine thousand wounded and completed the task within twelve hours—no easy accomplishment for the litter bearers because of Confederate sniper fire; because of the bitter cold, which for the wounded still lying on the field meant frosted and frozen limbs; and because of the short time in which the Union army had to retreat from its positions for fear of a counterattack by General Robert E. Lee. Although Union forces suffered defeat, they were able to evacuate their wounded from field hospitals on the south side of the Rappahannock River by December 15 and to remove all wounded to Washington by the twenty-fifth of December.[81]

On March 30, 1863, Grant approved General Orders No. 22, establishing a similar ambulance corps in the Army of the Tennessee. Experience in the field dictated certain changes, which became part of the revised *Regulations* published as General Orders No. 85 on August 24, 1863. In the spring of 1864, Congress formally established a uniform system of ambulance corps for the army based upon Letterman's regulations. Approved by the president on March 11, 1864, and promulgated by the secretary of war in General Orders No. 106 on March 16, 1864, the Ambulance Corps was placed under the control of the medical director of the army, combining elements of Larrey's *ambulance volante* and Percy's *brancardiers*. The orders furnished each army corps with ambulances, horse and mule litters, stretchers, and other appliances as prescribed by the medical director and the surgeon general. In addition, the medical director had complete control over a fixed number of men detailed on the basis of the ambulances and other wagons authorized to the organization. The act further prohibited any use of the ambulances except for hospital purposes, and no persons other than medical officers or those detailed to the ambulance were permitted to accompany sick or wounded to the rear.[82]

In the field, the medical director determined the number of ambulances and wagons that would accompany the troops, as well as the amount of hospital supplies, clothing, and rations to be put up in ambulance boxes. Stretchers went to the front strapped on the ambulances. When battle began, the director established field collection depots for the wounded at points most convenient for ambulances but close enough to the action to be effective. The medical director also selected sites for division hospitals, which, as a general rule, he "placed near the most practicable roads, in the rear of the centre of the troops, and sufficiently to the rear to be out of the ordinary range of the enemy's guns; suitable ground, good water, and plenty of fuel must of course decide the choice of locality." If overrun by enemy forces, the director made sure that the wounded received proper shelter and that sufficient medical officers, attendants, and medical supplies remained behind for their comfort. This latter action, which the Geneva Convention would later codify, reflected a practical humanitarian concern understood by combatants long before the signing of the Geneva Convention.[83]

The chief ambulance officer of a brigade moved with the troops to ensure that drivers and stretcher-bearers operated at their established posts. His duties involved maintaining the ambulances; making sure that drivers attended the horses; provisioning all water kegs; instructing stretcher-bearers; and, in action, ensuring that "wounded men are loaded carefully and speedily and the drivers do not get demoralized."[84]

When, by the summer of 1864, the Medical Department of the Army of the Potomac came under the leadership of Surgeon Thomas A. McParlin, who succeeded Letterman, the army had a department that had learned from its experiences and supported the sick and wounded with efficiency and dependability. Battle tested, the ambulance and field-hospital service designed by Letterman was so complete and practical that it soon became a model for field medical service in all of Europe's armies. The genius of both Hammond and Letterman resulted in a field-relief system that met the needs of wound emergencies on the field, ensured efficient evacuation of the wounded to field and fixed hospitals behind the lines, and achieved this in a manner that was both effective and adaptable to all modern armies.[85]

By April 1864, the Fifth Corps' Ambulance Corps and Train consisted of 17 commissioned officers of the line, 550 enlisted men, 171 two-horse ambulances, 62 supply wagons, 11 medicine wagons, 528 horses, and 348 mules. In the Wilderness campaign (May 5–6, 1864), the Army of the Potomac provided one ambulance for every 150 men, enabling Surgeon McParlin to carry out the plans of his predecessor effectively.[86] The surgeon directed that one-half of the ambulances follow the division on its march while the other half remain on call with the supply train. During the battle, the Union army was supported by aid stations, collecting stations, and ambulance stations established behind the brigades.[87]

Despite these improvements in ambulance organization, the U.S. Army still lacked sufficient organizational capability to link the field hospitals with the evacuation hospitals and to determine whether to treat a wounded man on the field, usually inadequately, or to delay treatment until the patient reached a place where medical intervention could be carried out under more favorable conditions. Unfortunately for the wounded, the work of Louis Pasteur and Joseph Lister came too late; Lister's work was not published until 1867. For the most part, the thirteen thousand physicians who served in the Union army and the thirty-two hundred who served the South practiced with old ideas and few new tools. The surgeon's field companion, devised in 1863 by Medical Inspector Richard H. Coolidge, replicated those designed by the British. It contained chloroform, extract of ipecac, ginger, persulfate of iron, whiskey, tincture of opium, compound cathartic pills, sulfate of quinine pills, opium pills, isinglass plaster, medicine cups, scissors, teaspoons, pins, thread, lint, toweling, bandages, muslin, and corks. Surgeons typically used chloroform as an anesthetic, followed by morphine or opium for pain. Physicians had available only a few stethoscopes, not more than a dozen thermometers, and probably even fewer syringes. Nevertheless, by the close of the war, the Union army had some 225 hospitals supporting its sick and wounded.[88]

In the Confederate army, an assistant surgeon and a detail of thirty infirmary corpsmen were assigned to care for a regiment's wounded on the field and to remove them to field infirmaries. Corpsmen were unarmed and wore special badges to distinguish them from the fighting soldier. Every two corpsmen had the responsibility for a litter, and each carried water, bandages, tourniquets, splints, and a bottle of brandy or whiskey as a stimulant. The infirmary corps replaced those troops who broke ranks to assist wounded comrades from the field. Although the Confederacy directed each regiment to have at least two ambulance wagons, with additional wagons in reserve, this seldom happened: its armies faced a chronic ambulance shortage. Few ambulances of any type were available, a situation that forced assistant surgeons to keep the wounded on the field, often under impossible conditions. While assistant surgeons worked on the field, surgeons remained at brigade or division infirmaries, performing essential surgical operations and directing the evacuation of wounded to general hospitals in the rear. The Confederacy resorted to all types of wagon transport and tried, whenever possible, to evacuate wounded to railroad depots or steamer landings for transport to hospitals in Richmond and other key cities.[89]

By the conclusion of hostilities, the enlistments in the Union army during the war totaled 2,898,304; because of incomplete records, the number of men in the Confederate armies can only be estimated at between six and eight hundred thousand. While they were at times faced with long periods of inactivity, armies on other occasions fought battle after battle in rapid succession, with their dead and wounded numbering in the tens of thousands. In the battle of Gettysburg alone, General George G. Meade reported fifteen thousand wounded; other battles showed similarly gruesome numbers. Although the figures provided by the adjutant general and by the surgeon general of the U.S. Army show slight differences in deaths from wounds and disease, the gross figures are consistent in their magnitude. By war's end, the total number of casualties on both sides would approximate a million men, while the estimated deaths from battle, disease, and accidents would amount to nearly six hundred thousand.[90]

The public and the military continued to debate the merits of the ambulance system throughout the war years, but an observer, writing in the *North American Review* in 1864, predicted that the nation would teach the Old World many lessons in the prosecution of war—lessons that went beyond the capacity for destroying the enemy.[91]

2

Early Ambulance Technology

Major Richard Delafield, reporting on his Crimean experiences, wrote: "The requisites for an ambulance should be such as to adapt to the battlefield, among the dead, wounded, and dying, — in ploughed fields, on hill-tops, mountain slopes, in siege batteries and trenches, and a variety of places inaccessible to wheel-carriages, of which woods, thick brush, and rocky ground are frequently the localities most obstinately defended." Given the variety of conditions, no single medical evacuation system applied to all occasions. Thus, soldiers, stretcher-bearers, and ambulance attendants found themselves continually challenged to assist the nonambulatory soldier with a combination of regular and extemporaneous methods.[1]

CAMEL LITTERS AND DANDIES

Throughout history, armies have employed horses, mules, oxen, camels, llamas, elephants, and humans to transport their wounded. In the corps of the Punjab Frontier Force in India, the common, or duree, dandy served the army's bearer needs. With poles of thick bamboo, sixteen feet in length, the dandy earned a reputation for transporting wounded on hilly terrain and for providing comfort to the patient over long marches. For the severely wounded, however, the British army preferred the stronger Bareilly dandy, which provided more comfort for fracture cases and for those with wounds of the chest and upper extremities, where the patient had to be carried in a sitting or upright position (plate 6). The dhoolie, on the other hand, was a closed-in litter carried by two or four bearers with two others in attendance. This carriage became the staple transport for the sick and wounded in England's Eastern wars. During campaigns in India, six hundred dhoolie bearers served a fighting battalion of one thousand. Although some advocates recommended the dhoolie for European conflicts, including the Crimean War, the military refused to approve their plans. Instead, dhoolies remained the standard transport only in areas of the world with large populations, as in the attack upon Canton in 1857 and in the Indian Mutiny of 1859.[2]

Camel litters provided transport in the 1830s and 1840s in British India and during the Afghan campaigns (plate 7). The term *litter* derived from the Latin *lectica*, meaning a form of couch or bed. Those servants who carried the bed were called *lecticarii*, or litter bearers. Indian natives gave the term *kujjawa* to this form of transport because it reminded them of a hamper used in Afghanistan to transport fruit long distances. Four men could travel upright in the camel litter, two horizontally. The frame included an awning and curtains, which shielded patients from the sun. During battle, the British army preferred camel litters to bearers, who were apt to flee. Medical officers also transported their wounded by this means to more distant towns or villages for recuperation. The British moved convoys of sick and wounded by camel kujjawa, which they considered more cost-effective than the dhoolie; however, because of its peculiar swaying motion, the British preferred to use the camel litter for convalescents rather than for the seriously sick and wounded.[3]

CACOLETS AND MULE LITTERS

After the medical evacuation problems encountered in the siege of Sebastopol in the Crimea, the English, French, and Sardinian armies adopted pack mules for carrying litters and cacolets. This experience, recounted by Major Richard Delafield in his *Report to the Senate* in 1860, resulted in his subsequent request for chairs and litters in the American Civil War. Delafield recognized that, given the sorry state of roads at the front and the congestion that often prevented the passage of ambulance wagons—first preference being given to artillery, ammunition wagons, reinforcements, and food—chairs and litters would minimize the problems of evacuating the wounded.[4] Accordingly, in May 1861, the Quartermaster's Department purchased mule litters and cacolets patterned after those used by the French army in Algeria and in the Crimean War. Tiffany and Company of New York and G. Kohler built the conveyances and purchased animals specially trained for the purpose. By July 1862, these companies had provisioned the Union army with three hundred mule litters and cacolets resembling those used in the Crimea (plate 8).[5]

Despite these purchases and Delafield's good intentions, efforts to introduce mule litters and cacolets at the battle of Fair Oaks (May 31 through June 1, 1862), proved futile, as did other efforts by the army in the Shenandoah Valley, under General Nathaniel P. Banks, and at the battle of Antietam. Horses proved too restless and mules too untrainable for effective use. The lack of trained animals and drivers available at the same place and time with the litters and cacolets meant that ambulance matériel designed and manufactured at considerable cost was never really tested in the field. Under battle conditions, armies tended to requisition available horses and mules for other services, particularly to carry munitions. Furthermore, the army objected to experimenting with the conveyances; many soldiers simply saw them as unnecessary baggage, a burden to transport, and obviously inconvenient during battle. Medical men and soldiers preferred hand litters improvised during the battle as the most appropriate and convenient means of transporting the wounded to ambulance stations or hospitals.[6] As Surgeon George Suckley, medical director of the Eleventh Corps of the Army of the Potomac, explained in a letter of March 20, 1863, to Surgeon J. H. Brinton, "There are no cacolets in this corps, and I want none. Three hundred and fifty pounds weight is too much for a mule's back over rough ground, encumbered by bushes, stones, logs and ditches. Among trees, cacolets will not answer at all; although used in European services and in Algeria, they have there been employed under some favorable circumstances, either on plains or on open rolling country. Here they would prove, I sincerely believe, only a troublesome and barbarous encumbrance, cruel alike to the wounded and the pack-animals."[7]

The effort to introduce cacolets proved to be an expensive waste of time. At a cost of twenty-one thousand dollars (not counting the purchase and training of mules), the cacolet experiment ended in failure; the quartermaster general could not demonstrate that even one wounded man was ever carried or that officers in the field showed a willingness to test the equipment. Instead, armies chose to rely on wheeled ambulances and hand litters. Mules originally purchased for the cacolets were eventually transferred to ambulances and general-purpose wagons.[8]

Although abandoned by the Union armies, unsuccessful in India during the Sepoy rebellion, and a failure in New Zealand during the Maori War in 1860, French cacolets and mule litters demonstrated their usefulness in the Italian War of 1859 and again in the Franco-Austrian invasion of Mexico in 1864–65. In 1865, the French in Algeria organized a light field hospital, or mule ambulance system, using cacolets for carrying the sick and wounded. For every thousand soldiers, the army provided eighteen mules with cacolets and a field hospital. Nevertheless, this system was not without problems. In the Mexican campaign, officers and men complained that the cacolets were unserviceable on narrow mountain passes, and horses and mules were unable to bear the weight of the wounded. The varying gaits of the animals intensified the discomfort of the injured, and the high center of gravity not infrequently caused the loss of both animal and soldier down a deep ravine.[9]

While armies continued to criticize mule litters and cacolets, they almost unanimously supported the stretcher as the best conveyance for the sick and wounded. During the American Civil War, the Union army issued 52,489 stretchers to its troops, approximately 25 per 1,000 men. By nineteenth-century standards, this liberal allocation, together with a supply of ambulance wagons, represented a magnitude "as had never been witnessed in any previous war." The stretchers were of different designs, beginning with the bulky and nonfolding Satterlee (named after Surgeon Richard S. Satterlee), or U.S. Regulation Army litter; followed by the Halstead folding stretcher, which, with minor modifications, continued in use through the 1880s.[10] The Satterlee weighed twenty-four and a half pounds and was twenty-seven inches wide; its poles, made of red ash and passing through a canvas bed, connected at either end to wrought-iron bands, which served as legs. The Schell litter, designed by Assistant Surgeon Henry S. Schell in 1862, was utilized as a bed in hospital tents. The eight-foot Halstead litter issued by the Medical Purveyor's Department connected to folding wooden legs fourteen and one-half inches long. This litter weighed nearly twenty-four pounds, detracting from its usefulness; moreover, the legs loosened over time, and its awkward structure inhibited use in ambulances, forcing bearers to remove the wounded soldier from the litter before placing him in the ambulance. Nearly thirteen thousand Halstead litters were furnished to troops during the Civil War. Its replacement, accepted by the army in 1895, was nine pounds lighter, folded compactly for easy carrying, and had fixed wrought-iron stirrup-shaped legs, which raised it four inches for transport in a regulation ambulance.[11]

At the Paris Exposition of 1867, M. Gauvin, a *medécin-major* in the French army, introduced a railcar spring stretcher that promised comfort during transport (plate 9). A year later, however, the Prussian government ordered railroads to utilize the ordinary field stretcher in transport, a decision based in large measure on the experiences of the Union army of the American Civil War. The only change introduced by the Prussian government was a folding backrest with different angles of elevation and two padded side pieces to prevent the recumbent patient from rolling off.[12]

The British employed a stretcher known as the Mark I and two later patterns devised by a Surgeon Major Faris known as Mark IV and Mark V. The Mark IV and V offered the advantage of wooden rollers, which facilitated their use in ambulances or other transport vehicles. Substitute stretchers included the hammock, used during the Ashanti War of 1874 and for shipboard transportation, and various extemporaneous stretchers, constructed of hay or straw rope, infantry straps and belts, or a combination of rifles and coats. Even telegraph wires served as useful substitutes for webbing between two stretcher poles or rifles, as did garments from an injured soldier, including vests, shirts, and trousers.[13]

WHEELBARROWS

One popular form of ambulance transport—used almost exclusively by Europeans—was the wheelbarrow, or hand wheel litter, designed with a single wheel and mounted with two support legs to provide stability. The wheelbarrow promised rapid removal of the wounded from battle while reducing the number of animals needed for transport service; it also lessened bearer fatigue. Instead of the two bearers required to carry a stretcher, a single attendant pushed a hand wheel litter. Although not recommended for long hauls, armies preferred the wheelbarrow for the short distance between where a soldier fell and the nearest surgical assistance.[14]

Larrey noted in his *Mémoires de chirurgie militaire, et campagnes* (1812–17) that he first used the wheelbarrow extensively in the summer of 1813 during the Russian campaign after the battle of Bautzen in Saxony. Upon Larrey's recommendation, bearers transported the wounded to Dresden in wheelbarrows owned by the local inhabitants. Filled with straw or small branches, a sack or a mattress, the carts adapted easily to ambulance transport.[15]

As a result of experiences in the Crimean War, Surgeon George Evans of London recommended the hand wheel litter that carried one wounded soldier in a recumbent position and another sitting. As an advantage, according to Evans, the litter also converted to an operating table in the field. Despite its versatility, the Board of Army Medical Officers in 1855 found it unacceptable. In 1860, England dispatched a number of two-wheeled ambulance barrows, litters, and cacolets to assist its forces in China. The so-called China ambulance (plate 10) served as a cart to carry provisions from the rear to the front and, by rearranging the rear board and sides, transformed from cart to ambulance. Unfortunately for its advocates, the popularity of river transportation prevented testing the full utility of the vehicle during the China campaign.[16]

In 1864, before the war with Denmark, Ignaz Josef Neudörfer (1825–98), an Austrian military surgeon and professor of surgery at the University of Prague, designed a two-wheeled litter after his experiences as medical officer of a field hospital during the Italian campaign in 1859 (plate 11). His conveyance, which he claimed could move easily over fields and rough terrain, was strong, light, inexpensive, and portable. The more successful Neuss two-wheeled litter, designed by government carriage builders in Berlin and constructed on principles similar to those of the Neudörfer, saw extensive use in the Austro-Prussian War against Denmark in 1864 (plate 12). In fact, during that war, a number of hand wheel carriages were specially constructed and tested. The favorable experience gained, particularly after the assault on the forts of Düppel, resulted in the development of many new wheeled conveyances intended to be powered by man. Proponents claimed that hand wheel litters ensured more rapid removal of the wounded than by ordinary stretchers; that they lessened the fatigue of bearers; that they avoided the necessity of using animals in bearing cacolets and mule litters; and that they were the preferred conveyance between the battle line and the first and second lines of surgical assistance. Nevertheless, Britain's Deputy Inspector General Thomas Longmore concluded that, while appropriate for war theaters with good roads, where the ground between the scene of battle and the lines of surgical assistance was clear and level, any other type of terrain required stretcher-bearers and mule transport.[17]

AMERICAN AMBULANCE WAGONS

Ambulance wagons designed specifically to support the sick and wounded did not exist in the United States prior to the establishment of the 1859 Medical Board. The army had attached no ambulances to its forces in the Florida war of 1838, the Mexican campaign of 1846–48, or the expeditions into Indian territories prior to the Civil War. What transport did exist consisted of improvised army wagons, oxcarts, and just about anything else available.

In 1858, an earlier board, consisting of surgeons Richard S. Satterlee and C. H. Lamb and Assistant Surgeon C. H. Crane, recommended the

Moses (named for Army Assistant Surgeon Israel Moses) for service in the West. This four-wheeled ambulance wagon, drawn by six horses or mules, looked like a cross between an omnibus and an ice cart. With entrance from the rear and two seats running lengthwise, it had a seating capacity of eighteen, with fourteen inside and an additional four on the front seat with the driver. At night, with the extension of a canvas shelter, it accommodated thirty men under its tentlike arrangement (plate 13). The board thought highly of the Moses design, considering it well suited for field and frontier service and for comfortable transport of the sick and wounded on long marches. Ironically, no action followed the board's recommendation, and apparently no Moses ambulances were built.

The two-wheeled Finley (named for Surgeon Clement A. Finley) and the two-wheeled Coolidge (for Assistant Surgeon Richard H. Coolidge) had springs and provided mattresses on the wagon floor. Both the Coolidge (plate 14) and Finley ambulances resulted from recommendations made by the 1859 board that ambulance transportation be furnished at the ratio of 40 men per 1,000 (twenty lying, twenty sitting) and that both two- and four-wheeled wagons were appropriate. In actual numbers, this meant one 2-wheeled ambulance to each company; one 4-wheeled and five 2-wheeled wagons to a battalion; and two 4-wheeled and ten 2-wheeled wagons to a regiment. The army sent these wagons to the military departments of Texas, New Mexico, Utah, California, and Oregon to test their capabilities. According to an observer in the *North American Review*, "no man who has once ridden in the two-wheeled ambulance would willingly get into one again, even if he were well." Soldiers referred to the two-wheeler as the "avalanche" because of the jarring ride it gave to the wounded. Even though the two-wheeled ambulance was touted as the best means for conveying the most seriously sick and wounded, the Union armies abandoned most of the two-wheelers by the second year of the war. According to Surgeon General Joseph K. Barnes, "their motion was intolerable and excruciating [and] wounded men begged to be taken out."[18]

In their place, the army relied upon the four-wheeled Tripler (named for Surgeon Charles S. Tripler), also recommended in 1859, which carried four litters (two tiers) and required four horses to pull it. The government produced the Tripler by the hundreds and used it throughout the Civil War (plate 15). The Tripler, ten feet long and four feet wide, held four spring mattresses (two lying on iron rails on the wagon bed and two hanging from the sides twenty-two inches above the floor); a chest of medicines and dressings; a front seat, which held three persons; and the tail of the carriage, which served as a seat for an additional three persons.

The entire carriage hung on platform springs to reduce jolting of patients.[19]

The most extensively used ambulance wagon during the Civil War was the Wheeling or Rosecrans (named for General William S. Rosecrans), weighing between seven and eight hundred pounds and furnished with padded seats, which accommodated eleven or twelve seated passengers or two in a recumbent position and two or three sitting (plate 16). Lighter than the Tripler and drawn by two horses, it had ample room for patients, water tank, extra litters, and medical supplies. While the body of the wagon rested on four elliptical springs, a soldier lying full length on the seat or bed of this four-wheeled ambulance "had to hold on with both hands to keep from falling to the floor," even on the reasonably smooth roads in Maryland. The experience was much worse in other areas of the war theater. But, lightweight, simple in construction, and easily repaired, the Wheeling survived the Civil War after participating in nearly every campaign and accompanied troops throughout the 1870s in the difficult terrain of the western service. Known affectionately as the "old yellow ambulance," the Wheeling elicited the support of faithful stalwarts and, around its tortured history, a host of stories—even folklore—developed. As a result, replacements for the Wheeling met with considerable skepticism.[20]

The four-wheeled Rucker (based on the design of Brigadier General Daniel H. Rucker), built toward the end of the Civil War by the government repair shops in Washington, provided large floor space, leather cushioned seats and backs, floor springs to support litters, and a box under the driver's seat for instruments, medicine chests, panniers, and other items. The Rucker (plate 17) carried two stretchers fitted with rollers to facilitate easy loading and unloading into the wagon. In addition, the ambulance could accommodate two additional stretchers suspended from the roof of the carriage. The body of the Rucker rested on platform springs, and its front wheels were smaller to improve turning radius. Although the ambulance weighed 1,120 pounds, outweighing the Wheeling by 450 pounds, it proved to be exceedingly durable compared to European designs. At the Paris Exposition of 1867, the U.S. Rucker, as modified by dentist Dr. Thomas Evans of Paris, who provided better ventilation, extra springs, and a rear seat, received one of the prizes offered for the best ambulance. Unlike many European designs that were lightweight and capable of carrying only a few wounded, the Rucker had an almost "democratic" appearance, was able to carry four litters, and was intended for rugged terrain and long distances.[21]

The Howard ambulance (named for Assistant Surgeon Benjamin Howard), constructed in October 1864, carried four recumbent patients and, as an innovation, the litters slid into the ambulance on rollers. It also provided a suspension arrangement to assist patients with fractured limbs. Although promising in its design, particularly with the use of semielliptical springs in place of the elliptical ones to reduce rolling and pitching, and the use of India-rubber blocks to reduce violent jarring, the Howard suffered from excessive weight (1,232 pounds) and chronic repair problems. Its only advantage seemed to be the convenience it provided for loading and unloading patients.

In the winter of 1864–65, the Fifth Army Corps Depot Hospital near Petersburg, Virginia, put into use an ambulance wagon (plate 18) designed by Dr. I. Langer that carried eight sitting or six sitting and two recumbent patients. It was little more than an army wagon refitted as an ambulance wagon, but it offered greater seating capacity, easy loading and unloading, and an apparatus for suspending two patients with thigh fractures. Following a review in April 1865, a board consisting of Colonel R. O. Abbott and Assistant Surgeons J. J. Woodward and William Thomson concluded that the Langer model was "ingeniously complicated" and therefore less useful than either the Wheeling or the Rucker wagon.[22]

By contrast, the Confederates had few ambulances. By 1863, the Confederate army in Mississippi could muster only thirty-eight wagons; and, by 1865, not one could be found in the entire brigade in the Department of West Virginia and East Tennessee. Instead, medical personnel improvised as well as they could, drawing upon army wagons and other transport.[23]

Following the war and after extensive and controversial tests involving a number of competing designs—including even an armored ambulance that converted into a portable rifle pit invented by H. N. Jasper—the 1878 Ambulance Board recommended a new vehicle known as the *McDermott*. Not until modified by a revised set of specifications, approved by Quartermaster General M. C. Meigs, did the ambulance win final approval and serve the Army Medical Department in the years between 1881 and 1892, when it was finally replaced by another model. The McDermott, known by many teamsters as "the mule killer" because of its excessive weight (fifteen hundred pounds), suffered from chronic brake problems, as well as a flawed wheel design that affected its ability to manage ruts. Nevertheless, the ambulance afforded ample floor space, leather cushioned seats and backs, lateral floor springs to support litters, and sufficient storage space to carry instruments, water, and other essentials. According to one historian, the McDermott "was a synthesis of the best features of American and European contemporary design." It was this ambulance that saw service in the post–Civil War army at Bear's Paw

Mountain, at the Powder River, and at instruction camps in the departments of Missouri, Platte, Dakota, and Arizona.[24]

Hospital Ships

During the Crimean War, England authorized the construction of specially designed ships to transport the sick and wounded. Among them, the *Andes* and *Cambria* provided hospital support for the Crimean Expeditionary Force by carrying wounded the three hundred miles across the Black Sea from the Crimea to Scutari. Two other ships, the *Bombay* and the *Mercia*, eventually joined in moving patients from Varna to Scutari. Later ships included the steamship *Kangaroo*, the sailing ship *Dunbar*, the *Avon*, the *Trent*, the *Sidney*, the *Pride of the Ocean*, the *Orient*, the *St. Hilda*, the *Robert Sale*, and the *William Jackson*. By the end of the war, forty or more ships of various kinds provided the British expeditionary force with the means for medical evacuation.[25]

Less than a decade later, during the American Civil War, the Union employed steamers for hospital service on the Mississippi River and on the Atlantic and Gulf coasts. In areas with available water transport, particularly on the Mississippi and its tributaries, hospital steamboats became a convenient method for moving the sick and wounded to base hospitals, as well as serving as receiving hospitals. Unfortunately for many of the wounded, the U.S. Sanitary Commission and the Quartermaster's Medical Department improvised their transport without much respect to comfort or condition of the vessel. As a result, complications from hospital gangrene occurred regularly due to the dampness and crowded conditions of the boats.[26]

In the eastern war theater, ship transport lacked hospital supplies of any sort, even mattresses. Some of the more noted ships included the *Daniel Webster*; the *Wilson Small*, which served as headquarters; and the *Elizabeth*, a small store boat that was fitted out by the Sanitary Commission. Other boats commissioned and staffed by the Sanitary Commission included the *S. R. Spaulding*, the *Knickerbocker*, the *Elm City*, the *State of Maine*, the *Enterpe*, and the *St. Mark*. This fleet of vessels carried sick and wounded to Fortress Monroe, Annapolis, and Washington. The *J. K. Barnes*, which went into active service in 1864, was assigned to the medical director of the Department of the South at Hilton Head Island, South Carolina. Over a year, she carried 3,655 patients, running mainly between Savannah, New Orleans, Charleston, and base hospitals in New York.[27]

In its efforts to move large numbers of wounded in the western theater, the Medical Department recognized the potential of boats fitted for hospital transportation. Such steamers as the *City of Memphis*, the *J. J. Roe*, the *War Eagle*, the *Crescent City*, and the *City of Louisiana* were chartered and fitted for carrying sick and wounded. The steamer *D. A. January* carried 12,299 sick and wounded over a period of seventeen months. Built in 1857 at Cincinnati, this side-wheeler carried patients from Pittsburg Landing, Tennessee; Paducah, Kentucky; and Helena, Arkansas; to St. Louis, Missouri; Keokuk, Iowa; New Albany, Indiana; and Cincinnati. Similarly, the steamboat *City of Louisiana* (later renamed the *R. C. Wood*) traveled 34,800 miles between April 1863 and April 11, 1865, making thirty-three trips, carrying 11,024 sick and wounded as it plied between New Orleans, Memphis, Vicksburg, St. Louis, and Louisville. Other steamers serving the western theater included the *City of Alton*, the *Ginnie Hopkins*, the *Empress*, the *Red Rover*, the *Imperial*, the *Stephen Decatur*, and the *J. S. Pringle*.[28]

The Cincinnati branch of the Sanitary Commission chartered the *Allen Collier*, a 133-ton stern-wheel steamer, stocking it with hospital supplies and supporting it with a staff of nurses and surgeons. Despite constant acrimony with the military, the commission supported the needs of the wounded when Fort Donelson fell to the Union forces of Commodore Andrew Hull Foote and General U. S. Grant in February 1862. Eighty-one of the Union and Confederate wounded were moved by steamer to hospitals at Cincinnati, Louisville, Paducah, Mound City, and St. Louis.[29]

Unfortunately, hospital steamers suffered one principal drawback. They carried not only the sick and wounded but an assorted list of stragglers. As one critic complained, the steamers had become the living space of

> all the friends of the sick and wounded [and] every man, woman, and child . . . impressed with the slightest inkling that their hearts contained one particle of sympathy for the poor soldier: curiosity seekers, sanitarians, state agents, sutlers, committees from various associations, one and all concluded they had a right to transportation of such a boat. This of course was out of the question, as it prevented the employees from properly cleaning the boat and took up room required for patients. More than this, it used up the subsistence which belonged to the hospital fund, which was used to buy so many things necessary for the diet of the sick. It was annoying to the surgeons, it was in the way of all discipline, and in fact disagreeable to every one.[30]

Throughout the course of the war, steamers were pawns in the continual strife between the Medical Department and the Quartermaster's Department. No sooner had the Medical Department fitted boats for hospital transport than the Quartermaster's Department claimed them for troop transport. When this occurred, the boats inevitably came back stripped of their furnishings, requiring costly refitting. Rancorous letters between the

Surgeon General's Office and the secretary of war noted this unfortunate situation and the desire of the Medical Department exclusively to control its boats. Not until February 1865 did the secretary of war agree to end the interference of the Quartermaster's Department and place control of the hospital transport steamers completely in the hands of the Medical Department.[31]

THE RAILROAD AS AMBULANCE

The expansion of railroads in the nineteenth century proved enormously important for the military, both in terms of rapid concentration of men, munitions, and stores and in terms of removing the sick and wounded. The development of trunk lines and their interlacing networks of feeders became essential elements in military planning. But, recognizing that railroads offered a possibility of speedy removal from the battle line did not come without differences of opinion. Military surgeons, fearing untimely delays, argued that severely wounded soldiers (i.e., those with shot fractures and those with wounds to the body cavity or to large joints) should be regarded as neutrals and treated as near the field of battle as possible. Nevertheless, the pressures for rapid removal prevailed as railroad transport promised to alleviate the harshness and suffering at the front lines and also to reduce the number of combatants required to attend the sick and wounded under critical battle conditions. Clearly, the wounded received better treatment at a base hospital away from the chaos of battlefield medicine. Their distribution to permanent hospitals far from the battlefield reduced the threat of contagion and other illnesses that frequented armies and decimated those already in weakened conditions.[32]

The earliest European test of rail capability for medical evacuation came in the Crimea with the five-mile railway from Balaclava to battery positions at the front. Although a locomotive hauled the eight-wagon train over the first two miles, the remainder of the trip was accomplished by a stationary engine for the steep incline and then horses.[33] Europe's armies also used the railroad as ambulance support at Châlons-sur-Marne in 1857; more extensive utilization occurred two years later in the Italian War of 1859 when the Austrian, French, and Sardinian armies employed passenger trains to transport their wounded to hospitals in Milan, Brescia, Pavia, and Turin. In all, eighty-nine thousand casualties were moved by rail during that conflict. Subsequently, French military surgeon M. Périer converted baggage cars for hospital transport, and Ernst J. Gurlt of Berlin made a similar proposal for carrying wounded in hammocks suspended from the panels of freight cars by iron hooks. Despite these early designs, armies undertook few improvements or special arrangements. Most of the wounded were simply laid on straw mattresses or directly upon loose straw that covered the floors of freight cars.

During the American Civil War, armies and private relief organizations tested the full potential of the railroad. Indeed, the war has often been called a "railway war," with military officers and civilians working together to adapt railroads to the strategic movements of troops. The railroad brought new mobility to armies, enabling commanders to move soldiers, horses, mules, artillery, and baggage long distances and to deploy them effectively and quickly against an enemy force. However, away from these iron roads, transportation remained as primitive as in the days of the American Revolution.[34]

The first occasion for conveying sick and wounded was in August 1861, following the battle of Wilson's Creek in central Missouri. After falling into enemy hands and then being paroled, the Union wounded collected at the southwestern terminus of the St. Louis Railroad at Rolla. There, the Union army requisitioned freight cars, fitted them for carrying the wounded, and then transported the wounded the 103 miles to St. Louis hospitals. Medical officers also experimented with various extemporaneous methods for carrying the seriously wounded in freight cars, including suspending litters from poles attached to the floor and roof (a variation of the Zavodovsky system) and building wooden bunks filled with straw. In most of these cars, workers also improvised windows by sawing out spaces in the walls to improve ventilation.[35]

The Union army drew its ambulance railcars from several different sources. It requisitioned the greatest number from empty supply trains stationed at depots close to the war theater; others it drew from worn-out or condemned freight or passenger cars purchased secondhand and then altered (plate 19) to carry the sick and wounded. And, when available, the military (or the Sanitary Commission) built hospital cars from new operating stock. By the end of the war, the North had moved 225,000 of its sick and wounded by rail from the war theater to general hospitals in the rear.[36]

The Bureau of Construction of Military Railways, the surgeon general, and the United States Sanitary Commission prepared specifications for this special rolling stock. Assistant Superintendent of Military Railroads J. McCrickett designed the hospital cars on the Orange and Alexandria Railroad, which ran between the army's encampment near Culpeper, Virginia, and base hospitals at Alexandria and Washington. The car, forty-five feet in length, transported patients in both stretchers and chairs. McCrickett arranged the stretchers in three tiers, the first tier consisting of permanent couches with mattresses, and the second and third tiers of field stretchers suspended by metal, rubber, or leather straps secured to pegs inserted in permanent poles. The car accommodated those less sick or wounded by having them sit on couches and assigning others to lie on the second- and third-tier litters.[37]

The railroad became a vital part of the transport system when the theater of war moved into Maryland and Pennsylvania. More than nine thousand sick and wounded moved over the Aquia Creek Road following the battle of Chancellorsville (May 2–4, 1863). In the aftermath of Gettysburg (June 27 to July 4, 1863), the army transported more than fifteen thousand men from field hospitals to Baltimore, New York, Harrisburg, and Philadelphia. In most instances, boxcars from returning supply trains served as the vehicles of transport, with stretchers placed on floors covered with hay to cushion the jarring motion of the trains. Each car contained a watercooler, tin cups, bedpans, and other essentials. The Philadelphia and Reading Railway Company fitted freight cars using the same stretchers that supported patients in the ambulance wagons. Cars constructed on this basis contained fifty-one berths, with a seat at each end for an attendant.[38]

By 1864, three hospital trains, each consisting of ten to twelve cars and fitted under the supervision of Surgeon George E. Cooper, medical director of the Department of the Cumberland, and Surgeon O. O. Herrick of the Thirty-fourth Illinois Volunteers, connected the advance army with base hospitals in Louisville. The trains had cars for carrying casualties, several baggage cars, one car fitted as a kitchen, another as a dispensary, and accommodations for a medical officer. In this manner, wounded men moved the 175 miles from Nashville, Tennessee, to Louisville, Kentucky.[39]

Another hospital car, designed by physician Elisha Harris (1824–84) and built by the Sanitary Commission, provided a gangway through the center of each carriage. Quartermaster General Meigs placed all cars at the government depot at Alexandria under Harris's disposal. There, in cooperation with the three railway companies owning the line between Washington and New York, Harris prepared his cars. Using India-rubber tugs, he suspended three tiers of beds, sixteen of which swung along each side of the hospital car. Those soldiers able to sit filled invalid chairs and broad couches. By 1862, Harris hospital cars were running daily between Marietta, Georgia, and Louisville.[40] Daily, at least one train left the vicinity of the field hospitals for the trip to the base hospitals. Its yellow flag with green border, three red lanterns, and bright scarlet smokestack were recognized symbols, respected by the Confederate army, which allowed it to proceed while seizing or wrecking other trains. These ambulance trains traveled unmolested, with orders from Confederate General Nathan B. Forrest and Colonel John Morgan not to interfere with their purpose. Until William Tecumseh Sherman's march to the sea, the trains ran regularly from the front to base hospitals four hundred miles distant.[41]

In 1864, the Union army established a base depot hospital at the junction of the James and Appomattox rivers in Virginia. The depot became the center for transport to hospital steamers and other hospital or recuperation centers. Most troops transported to the depot arrived in boxcars, which had originally carried supplies to the theater of war. Although designed to accommodate nine to ten recumbent patients, each car typically carried twenty wounded. Lack of hay and straw meant that the wounded frequently had to lie on bedding made of dry leaves or evergreen boughs. The army eventually converted a number of passenger cars by erecting rows of stanchions from which they suspended litters. The suspension system carried a certain risk: jolting over poorly laid rails occasionally caused litters to break from their connecting rings.[42]

In the West, a similar system of rail ambulances proved equally effective. Although transportation remained within the jurisdiction of the Quartermaster's Department, the Sanitary Commission continued to urge the transfer of the management function to the Medical Department.[43]

The Confederate army provided no regular system of hospital trains, relying instead upon extemporaneous methods in passenger cars, freight cars, and open boxcars. Dr. Samuel Preston Moore, surgeon general of the Confederate army, recalled in 1875 that "freight and open box cars were used to transport our wounded from the field to the hospitals. The cars were bedded with straw or leaves, whichever was most convenient. The method was found to be objectionable on account of the bedding becoming foul and unpleasant and was discontinued and blankets were placed on the floor when they could be procured." Lacking rubber rings to suspend litters in the manner devised by Elisha Harris, the Confederates substituted ropes fastened to posts.[44]

Perhaps the most important ambulance innovation of the war was the use of the same stretcher that carried the wounded man from the field of battle as transport on the railroad and support for the soldier upon his arrival at the base hospital. For this and other innovations, military surgeon Johannes Friedrich August von Esmarch (1823–1908), professor at Kiel, remarked that "the U.S. Federal Government, which, at the instigation of the world-renowned Sanitary Commission, organized the transport of wounded on railways so perfectly as to leave little to be desired, might well serve as an example to European States in future wars."[45]

Besides the American Civil War, the railroad was used for medical evacuation in the Schleswig-Holstein War of 1864, the Austro-Prussian-Italian conflict of 1866, the Franco-Prussian War of 1870–71, and the Serbian-Bulgarian War of 1885–86. During the Franco-Prussian War, Germany moved its wounded to the nearest railhead for immediate transport to hospitals situated near the frontier, thus eliminating the need for field hospitals. Britain used railways in the Zulu War of 1879, the Boer rebellion of 1881, the Egyptian campaigns of 1884 and 1885, Rhodesia in 1896, and the Sudan in 1898. The railroad also played an important role in the Turco-Greek War of 1897, the Boer War of 1899–1902, the Russo-Japanese War of 1904, and the Balkan War of 1912–13.

NATIVE AMERICAN TRAVOIS

The origin of the travois is obscure. Francis Parkman, in his *History of the Conspiracy of Pontiac, and the War of the North American Tribes Against the English Colonies After the Conquest of Canada* (1851), described how North American Indians transported their sick and wounded by a conveyance of poles fastened to each side of a pony; the ends dragged along the ground, and between the poles stretched animal hides. During the war with Pontiac in 1763, colonists quickly adopted the conveyance to transport their own wounded. Within decades, Lewis and Clark (1804–6) and medical officers on many frontier posts had copied the technique.[46]

Army medical officers made frequent use of the Indian travois and its imitations. Hastily contrived hammocks; pack animals, equipped with sacks of stuffed straw, leaves, or grass; and pallets of hay or straw served the emergency needs of soldiers in improvised situations (plate 20). During the Florida campaigns against the Seminole Indians in 1835–36, for example, Surgeon Richard S. Satterlee improvised a system for transporting wounded soldiers using litters made from blankets and hides of cattle strung between horses. During the same Florida campaign, Captain H. L. Thistle of the Louisiana Volunteers designed a single-horse litter for transporting wounded. Years later, during the war with Mexico (1846–48) and the expedition against the Apache Indians in 1852, the army employed a two-horse litter not unlike that described by Randolph B. Marcy in his *Prairie Traveler. A Handbook for Overland Expeditions* (1859). The double-mule litter remained a popular form of transport for the sick and wounded during the Indian campaigns of the 1870s. The cavalry used it in mountainous terrain and in other off-road engagements (plate 21). In typical situations, the poles were connected to a network of ribbing over which a soldier spread a buffalo robe, blankets, and pillows. Often, the rawhide used for the ribbing came from the skins of dead horses or ponies.[47]

Concern for the transport of the sick and wounded led the military Medical Board of 1859 to recommend that the two-horse litter be issued to frontier posts in the West. The army incorporated this litter, a prototype of which saw action in the earlier campaigns in Florida and Mexico, into the 1861 revision of army *Regulations*. The army continued to rely upon the two-horse litter as late as 1873, with improvised variations continuing into the Second World War. According to the *Regulations*, the army allotted 40 litters per 1,000 troops in those areas where two-wheeled carriages proved inappropriate or were unavailable. These litters consisted of two poles, constructed in sections extending sixteen feet in length and connected to a canvas bed.[48]

The Native American travois became the basis for the Greenleaf, Cleary, Girard, and McDougill travoises constructed by the army. The McDougill travois, invented by Captain Thomas M. McDougill, U.S.A., consisted of two poles eighteen feet in length, which supported a canvas bed strengthened by metal rods to form a horizontal litter. The Greenleaf travois, designed by Lieutenant Colonel Charles R. Greenleaf, deputy surgeon general, U.S.A., transported the sick and wounded when wheeled vehicles proved impractical. The apparatus could be packed into a bundle nine feet long and one foot in diameter for portability.[49] The horse litter proposed by Assistant Surgeon Peter A. J. Cleary, U.S.A., originated from his experiences and observations at Fort Still in the Indian Territory in 1875.[50]

Following the battle of Little Big Horn (June 25, 1876) in Montana, the army transported nineteen severely wounded soldiers on the two-mule litters, ten on travoises, and thirty on horseback. Four men attended each mule litter, one leading the forward mule, one the rear mule, and one on either side of the litter to steady its swaying movement. In spite of these precautions, the mules that the army had recovered from General George Armstrong Custer's pack team were skittish and, on at least one occasion, threw a wounded soldier from his litter.[51]

Overall, the military found the travois more useful than the two-mule litter because of its easier construction, the fewer animals and men required for support, and the scarcity of poles for carrying the wounded. In rough terrain, soldiers carried the ends of the travois over obstructions while allowing it to drag over smooth ground. As an added benefit, weakened patients were less likely to fall from the supports.

The McElderry single-mule litter (plate 22), designed for broken country, was used in the actions against the Modoc Indians in the lava beds of southern Oregon and northern California in 1872 and 1873. According to its inventor, Assistant Surgeon H. McElderry, the litter required little training of mules, which was important because the army almost always organized its litter trains extemporaneously from pack animals released to a medical officer.[52]

Despite efforts to improve ambulance support, Surgeon John Moore, U.S.A., recalled that troops in the late 1870s generally disregarded horse litters and cacolets when on the move. He remembered few instances of their actual use; rarely were soldiers so removed from ambulance wagons or wheeled supply vehicles that they were forced to depend upon the litter or cacolet for transportation.[53]

Like the Civil War's experiments with the cacolet, efforts to provide cavalry in the western service with the Rooker saddle attachment (designed by W. B. Rooker) proved hopelessly futile (plates 23, 24). Experiments in 1875 and 1876 in Wyoming and the Dakotas failed to elicit the support of either officers or men. Although the army provided Rooker saddle attachments at Fort Brown, Texas; at Fort Laramie, Wyoming; and at Fort Leavenworth, Kansas; as well as with army expeditions in Arizona and Utah, soldiers preferred to carry as little baggage as possible and, in treating their wounded or sick, found their own extemporaneous methods preferable to the Rooker attachment.[54]

MEDICINE WAGONS

During the early months of the Civil War and in the western service, the army typically transported its medicines in ordinary supply or ambulance wagons and in panniers carried by pack animals. Not until March 1862 did Surgeon Jonathan Letterman provide instructions for the construction of a special medicine wagon for close support of the military. The army eventually provided each brigade with a wagon furnished with stores, dressings, furniture, appliances, and an amputating table. Exemplifying the various types of wagons used in the Civil War were the Dunton regimental medicine wagon, the Perot medicine wagon, and the Autenrieth pattern (plate 25), first used during the last year of the war. The Dunton wagon, proposed in November 1862, opened on the sides to dispense medicines. The Autenrieth medicine wagon, recommended by the Medical Board (Surgeons C. H. Crane, R. O. Abbott, and Charles Sutherland), was constructed by the government shops and adopted during the last year of the war.[55]

The need for more rapid transport became apparent during the Indian wars, when emergencies faced by small forces, such as scouting parties, required ambulance and medical assistance without the encumbrance of the larger wagons designed for brigades. In the Powder River expedition against the Sioux in 1876, for example, the army carried its medical supplies on two-pack mules (plate 26). The supplies consisted of a valise of surgical equipment, including instruments, dressings, and chloroform; a medicine pannier; two cases carrying twelve blankets each; a rubber bedcover; and bottles of brandy. Additional materials included an amputating knife, ball forceps, artery forceps, and beef extract.[56]

The army also authorized the construction of a one-horse, two-wheeled transport cart (plate 27) for hospital supplies. The Watervliet Arsenal in West Troy, New York, constructed the cart and delivered it to the Surgeon General's Office in Washington in January 1876. The cart carried three chests designed to hold surgical instruments, medicines, hospital stores, mess furniture, and utensils. Each chest consisted of fitted trays containing spaces and compartments for individual appliances and medicines. The medical transport cart became an important addition to army field equipment.[57]

Overall, ambulance technology and organization labored to keep pace with the needs of the military through the first three-quarters of the nineteenth century. During those years, the industrial revolution acted as catalyst to inventors and manufacturers as they sought to make the best of mule- and horse-driven conveyances and the newer locomotive and steam-driven vessels. In large measure, battlefield medicine and its evacuation systems followed the chronicle of nationalism, wars, and imperial drives as nations flexed their muscles on behalf of unification or expansionist dreams. Only in the last quarter of the century did small-arms technology and long-range artillery take on such dimensions of destructive power as to challenge existing evacuation systems. Until then, ambulance technology remained relatively stable within the parameters of accepted warfare.

PART TWO

Consolidation

3

A World in Transition

By the mid-nineteenth century, the order that Metternich had imposed on Europe seemed to prevail in all corners and capitals. Indeed, the map of Europe in 1850 was not much different from the one the victors had drawn at Vienna in 1815. Nevertheless, neither Europe nor America was quite the same. The success of nascent nationalism and the emergence of Italy and Germany as nations profoundly changed the characteristics and behavior of European politics. The young American republic, while energetically expansionist, faced tortuous self-doubt regarding the nature and character of its growth. When its Civil War ended, the victorious North embarked on an economic and expansionist era of consolidation. In Europe, however, the sympathy to nationalism and economic expansionism came face-to-face with French interest, which clearly feared the implications of a consolidated middle Europe. The resulting tension between Napoléon III and the efficient Prussian military machine and the consequences for the future that the emergence of Germany as a united country meant for the powers of Europe determined the course of Europe's destiny and was a powerful contributing force to the eventual outbreak of the Great War.

DUNANT AND THE RED CROSS

In 1859, the Sardinian forces of Victor Emmanuel, with the allied army of France under Napoléon III, waged war against Austria for the liberation of northern Italy. Learning from their tragic experiences in the Crimea, the French adopted a plan that distributed their sick and wounded among a number of small hospitals in an effort to reduce the incidence of typhus and other infectious diseases. The Austrians, however, not as mindful of the Crimean debacle, were unprepared to support their forces when drawn into war against the superior Franco-Sardinian armies. After the battle of Magenta (June 4, 1859), more than eight thousand Austrian soldiers crowded into hospitals meant to accommodate only four thousand, resulting in unnecessary deaths from gangrene, typhus, and other diseases. In Verona, Nubra-Sima, Palma Nuova, and elsewhere, the oppressive heat and lack of transportation, shelter, and essential medical support resulted in high mortality. While the war in Italy demonstrated the effectiveness of the telegraph (as did the Crimea and the American Civil War), it also showed the need for transporting sick and wounded men by any available conveyance from field stations to more distant hospitals.

On June 24, 1859, Swiss philanthropist Jean-Henri Dunant (1828–1910), traveling to Lombardy to discuss his agricultural plans for Algeria with Napoléon III, came upon the final fifteen-hour battle of Solferino involving more than three hundred thousand men on a ten-mile front. There, he saw sixteen thousand French and Sardinian soldiers and twenty thousand Austrians left dead or wounded on the battlefield. For days after the battle, soldiers remained unattended and unburied where they had fallen. Appalled by this neglect, Dunant abandoned his business concerns and immediately threw himself into organizing relief efforts in Castiglione, calling upon volunteers to assist the thousands who otherwise seemed forgotten. For eight days, he directed relief in the villages around the battlefield and set about collecting linen and shirts, chamomile for washing wounds, lemons, sugar, and tobacco. Following the war, he became so obsessed with the horrors of what he had seen that, with the help of friends, he published his now-famous pamphlet *Un Souvénir de Solferino* (1862), which graphically depicted the aftermath of the battle.[1]

Besides telling the story of Solferino, Dunant urged the formation of volunteer relief societies to aid the sick and wounded in future battles. He also invited nations to recognize the universal principle of this humanitarian effort, to establish permanent societies of volunteer medical workers, and to respect organizations dedicated to that purpose. The publication of Dunant's work came at an auspicious moment. Building upon a genuine humanitarian concern for past military debacles, his idea stirred the conscience of European sovereigns and statesmen and acted as a catalyst for a conference to establish a voluntary international relief society. Dunant's forceful persuasion, along with the encouragement and support of Gustav Moynier, president of the Society of Public Utility; physicians Louis Appia and Theodore Maunoir; and General Guillaume-Henri Dufour, head of the Swiss federal forces, resulted in a meeting on February 9, 1863, and the establishment of a five-member committee titled the Permanent International Committee of Aid to Wounded Soldiers. General Dufour acted as chair of the committee, Dr. Moynier as vice-chair, and Dunant as secretary.[2]

The February 9 meeting resulted in a decision to form permanent relief societies for wounded soldiers throughout Europe and to organize a peacetime corps of volunteer nurses. Another consequence of this meeting (and of visits by Dunant to various European capitals) was a call for an international convention at Geneva during the summer of 1864. Preparatory to this convention, a preliminary conference of delegates from fourteen nations met in Geneva (October 26–29, 1863) and decided to support the establishment of committees of relief in all countries, the neutralization of personnel caring for the wounded, and the neutralization of the wounded themselves. The conference also adopted a distinctive red cross on a white armband as the badge of the volunteer medical personnel: the Red Cross.

After the October conference and prior to the meeting of delegates at the international convention, the permanent committee sent representatives to Schleswig to seek acceptance by the combatants in the Danish War (1864) of the principles adopted earlier at Geneva and to establish first-aid services for the wounded. This war, spurred by Otto von Bismarck's interest in the potential naval base of Kiel and by the pretext of protecting the rights of German nationals in Schleswig and Holstein, resulted in a crushing defeat for the Danes and the surrender of the duchies of Schleswig, Holstein, and Lauenburg to Austria and Prussia in the definitive Peace of Vienna, October 30, 1864.

From August 8 to 22, 1864, sixty-two delegates from sixteen nations (Baden, Belgium, Denmark, England, France, Hesse, Holland, Italy, Norway, Portugal, Prussia, Saxony, Spain, Sweden, United States, and Württemberg) met at Geneva. In addition, the Confederation of German States sent individual delegates to represent their members. Although Russia sent a delegation, it arrived too late to participate in the negotiations. On August 22, eleven governments signed the Convention of

Geneva, accepting formal rules for the organization and neutralization of hospitals and ambulance corps in times of war. The Geneva Convention stipulated that wherever its flag flew—over a wagon or a building—the area so identified was neutral. Unfortunately, the neutralization of the wounded was not clearly specified. The signatories agreed that all medical personnel aiding the sick and wounded would wear a white armlet bearing the distinctive Red Cross badge. The convention chose its red and white colors to compliment the Swiss republic, site of the first convention and home of its international headquarters. The convention simply reversed the red and white colors of the Swiss flag to create on a white background the Red Cross. As one historian noted, "Its similarity to the flag of the Swiss Confederacy, whose colours it simply reverses, was an intentional act of esteem for the little land that had supported the Cause in so exemplary and disinterested a way."[3]

The Red Cross movement was not without its critics, including the formidable Florence Nightingale, who feared that a voluntary, neutral international system would remove responsibility from governments and would weaken the military character of existing organizations. Each government, she argued, should be responsible for its own sick and wounded. What Nightingale failed to appreciate was that the intent of the originators of the convention was not to weaken governmental and military responsibility but rather to support it in a close, subordinate association.[4]

The Geneva Convention authorized the formation of a permanent international relief committee with headquarters in Geneva and established a plan for the formation of national relief societies. Gustav Moynier became the first president of the International Red Cross Committee and later president of the Swiss republic. Although the convention resulted in the creation of an international organization, the relief societies themselves were national, independent, and self-governing. Examples included the Johannritter Order of Germany, the Maltese Knightly Order of Germany, the Deutsche Ritter of Austria, the Order of St. John of Jerusalem in England (first established during the Crusades and reestablished in 1831, nearly three hundred years after its suppression by Henry VIII), and the Austrian Langue of the Sovereign Order of the Knights of St. John. Other organizations included the *Comité Central Belge*, the *Société Grecque de Secours aux Blessés* of Greece, the Central Italian Committee of the Red Cross, the *Comité Central de la Société Néerlandais de la Croix-Rouge*, and the *Comité Central Russe de la Croix-Rouge*.[5]

The signatories agreed to the notion of leaving the more seriously wounded behind as armies fell back after a battle. In doing so, the convention reversed the procedures of most field manuals, which urged that armies evacuate the more serious casualties first. "When it is remembered that every wounded man left to the enemy becomes a prisoner of war, and that all the Geneva Convention does for him is to ensure proper medical care and treatment till he recovers," commented William G. Macpherson in the *Journal of the Royal Army Medical Corps* in 1909, "it is evident that the chief concern of a commander in the field is to save as many wounded from capture as possible, and, above all, to save those who are likely to be able to return to the ranks in the shortest possible time." Thus, when armies chose to retreat from the field, officers first removed the less seriously wounded and only then evacuated the more severe cases. This change in policy allowed the ambulance corps to attend to the wounded, even after the withdrawal of their own army. By the Geneva agreement, armies regarded medical corpsmen as neutral and allowed them to return to their original division or unit.[6]

Following the Danish campaign of 1864, relations between Austria and Prussia fell apart when Bismarck proposed a federal reform in the Frankfurt Diet that excluded Austria. The war that quickly followed lasted seven weeks (June–August 1866) and was fought in three theaters: Italy, where the Italians were defeated on both land and sea; Germany, where General Vogel von Falkenstein and his army of fifty thousand defeated the Hanoverians at Langensalza; and Bohemia, where Helmuth von Moltke (using the lessons of the telegraph and the railroad from the American Civil War) advanced in three armies against the Austrians. At the decisive battle of Königgrätz (Sadowa) on July 3 in Bohemia, Prussian infantry, which had the advantage of the breech-loading "needle-gun," were able from their prone positions to decimate the standing Austrians using muzzle-loaders.

After the battle of Königgrätz, Prussian field hospitals faced the horrendous responsibility of caring for some thirty thousand wounded. This unexpected strain on men and equipment resulted in tragic outbreaks of cholera, pyemia, and hospital gangrene. Nearly half of those operated on died of their wounds or of subsequent infection. Although surgeons had introduced ether and chloroform anesthesia as early as 1847, surgical antisepsis did not become a part of Prussian military surgery until 1867. Doctors still regarded such instruments as the stethoscope (1819), syringe (1845), and clinical thermometer (c. 1860) as curiosities and did not fully integrate them into military medicine until the 1870s. Thus, in the battlefield environment, sepsis, wound infection, gangrene, tetanus, and erysipelas continued to take thousands of victims.[7]

The brevity of the war came as a surprise to Moynier and others within the Red Cross organization. Moreover, the failure of Austria and several of the German states to sign the Geneva Convention created considerable consternation despite Prussia's declared adherence without restriction. Dunant, acting as an intermediary and using what influence he could muster from the French and from Queen Olge of Württemberg, obtained Austrian adherence shortly after Königgrätz. This was soon followed by a July 9 order by Prince Alexander of Hesse, commander of the south German armies, to observe the Geneva Convention. With these breakthroughs, volunteer nurses demonstrated the practical and organizational abilities of the Red Cross.

In the early years following the Geneva accord, many held the mistaken belief that any person wearing the Red Cross badge could travel freely within the war zone without regard for military restrictions. Complicating this impression, many individuals wore Red Cross armbands while also carrying weapons, and Red Cross flags flew over shelters for the wounded that the armies also used for military purposes. According to John Furley, who served as director of the Ambulance Department of the Order of St. John (St. John Ambulance Brigade) in the Franco-Prussian War, "No badge has ever been more generally abused, both in peace and war, than the Red Cross." Furley insisted that the Red Cross was a military and not a civilian badge, and, "from a military point of view, no person is authorized to use it without official authority." By implication, Furley took issue with those Red Cross corps in the British army and elsewhere who occasionally carried arms.[8]

To protect the neutrality of those wearing the Red Cross, Furley insisted that the Geneva signatories strictly follow the stated purposes and uses of the badge. Anything less endangered innocent and neutral parties in a conflict. Thus, wagons requisitioned for carrying both ammunition and wounded could not carry a Red Cross flag. In fact, any effort to mask a military operation under the guise of the flag jeopardized those whose lives should otherwise be protected. Unfortunately, there existed no legal or punitive measure under convention rules to enforce proper use of the emblem, resulting in a form of behavior that included, among other things, the adoption of the badge by vendors of patented foods and medicines.[9]

Despite impediments, the rationality of the convention's articles prevailed; and, by the end of 1866, twenty nations adhered to the convention. Russia followed in 1867, and in 1868 the Papal States signed. Fearing "entangling alliances," the United States had steadfastly refused to sign the Geneva treaty. The efforts of Clara Barton, Charles S. P. Bowles (American delegate to Geneva), and Henry W. Bellows of the United States Sanitary Commission notwithstanding, it seemed to most

Americans that the Monroe Doctrine prohibited such involvement. Shortly before President James A. Garfield's assassination, Barton founded the American Association of the Red Cross (August 1881), which gave its first practical demonstration of relief during forest fires of that year in Michigan. When Chester A. Arthur became president, Barton entreated him to sign the agreement. On March 1, 1882, Arthur signed the Geneva treaty, making the United States the thirty-second signatory to the International Red Cross Society.[10]

By 1896, thirty-seven national Red Cross Societies had dedicated themselves to the support of the sick and wounded in time of war. And to ensure their readiness, most of these societies offered assistance during accidents, epidemics, and disasters affecting civilians. In 1899 at The Hague Peace Conference, the convention articles were extended to apply neutrality to wounded sailors as well as to ships and personnel providing their relief.[11]

THE FRANCO-PRUSSIAN WAR

The Franco-Prussian War (July 1870 to September 1, 1871) marked the culmination of Austria's defeat in 1866, the formation of the North German Confederation, and Bismarck's long-planned scheme to unify Germany. The change in Europe's balance of power without guaranteed compensations on the left bank of the Rhine and in Belgium proved unacceptable to France. Prussia's rejection of French demands, combined with mounting German nationalism and an aroused French public opinion, culminated in a war that both belligerents interpreted as the most appropriate vehicle for national policy. Soon after the war began, an outpouring of sympathy arose for the killed and injured on the field of battle, as well as for the countless thousands widowed, orphaned, and made homeless by the devastation. As a result, a number of countries joined in missions of mercy as both sides accepted volunteer help for the wounded.

With the outbreak of the war, the British National Society for Aid to Sick and Wounded (National Red Cross Society in England), composed largely of members of the Order of St. John, formed under the patronage of Queen Victoria and Edward, Prince of Wales. By the end of the conflict, British surgeons and nurses, equipped and supported by volunteer contributions, served in both the French and German armies. The English contingent of the National Society for Aid to Sick and Wounded, which offered its services to the French, faced war hysteria and the constant threat of imprisonment as spies. Another group of volunteers, known as Bart's Men, included Charles Mayo, M.D., who had earlier served in the

American Civil War. This group of the British Red Cross served the Prussian army and aroused great interest with their use of hypodermic syringes.[12]

During the conflict, the British National Society for Aid to Sick and Wounded had the opportunity to compare its own ambulance equipment with that of the combatants and of other volunteer groups. Most observers recognized Prussia's superior conveyances. The British sick-transport wagon, for example, which the members of the society used extensively in the war (plate 28), drew special criticism. Drawn by two horses and tested on the main roads of France, as well as in difficult terrain, the wagon proved excessively heavy and unduly harsh on horses, requiring additional animals to reduce the load. Subsequent recommendations included lighter construction, smaller front wheels to allow the wagon to turn more easily, a stronger roof, and the addition of a water barrel.[13]

At the request of American citizens living in Paris, Surgeon James Marion Sims (1813–83) headed an ambulance corps that supported the French army in the field. Almost immediately, however, differences of opinion arose between the sponsoring committee and the American surgical team, the former insisting that the surgeons and their medical supplies remain in Paris to await the anticipated coming of the German army. As a result of this schism within the American committee, the surgeons formed an alliance with the English, known as the Anglo-American Ambulance, and moved its services immediately to Sedan. The Americans included physicians Pratt, May, Tilghman, Nicoll, Hayden, Wallis, and Harry Sims. In all, there were eight Englishmen and eight Americans, with Marion Sims and William MacCormac sharing command.[14]

The Anglo-American Ambulance party located at Caserne d'Asfeld on the eve of the battle of Sedan. After the battle, with Marshal Marie-Maurice de MacMahon wounded and the French army suffering seventeen thousand casualties, Sedan capitulated. According to British correspondent Archibald Forbes, "We saw where MacMahon lay wounded and also how full the town was of troops. They were swarming, densely packed, everywhere. Of the wounded, some were in churches, the houses, public buildings and others lying unheeded and jostled in the courtyards: the dead were everywhere—in the gutters trampled on by the living, in the swampy margins of the moat, littering the narrow way through the glaces and the fortifications, lying some of them on the steps of the church, the sight was one never to be forgotten."[15]

The combatants on both sides of the conflict incorporated the principles of the Geneva Convention. Each of the national Red Cross societies developed rules and procedures, as modified by the military in whose area they operated. In some instances, the relationship worked without incident; in other situations, there were chronic difficulties. As a result of their experiences, Marion Sims and other American volunteers criticized the French medical evacuation system as cumbersome and unsuited for the realities of war.

The Prussian War Department had learned much from Larrey and Letterman as it had organized its mobile sanitary formations. The Prussian army employed companies of bearers, first introduced in 1855, who were distinguished by a special uniform and assigned to collect the wounded during battle and to carry them to dressing and field hospitals. The use of these companies prevented men from leaving the fighting ranks to carry comrades to the rear. In addition to the bearer companies, the army provided four auxiliary sick-bearers formed out of each company. These auxiliary bearers wore the uniform of their regiments but had a distinguishing badge on their left arm when serving as bearers.

To evacuate the wounded, German officers led the litter-bearer companies directly into the battle lines where they collected the wounded, gave first aid and refreshment, and conveyed them to ambulance wagons assembled at specified collecting stations to carry them to main dressing stations; from there they were taken to field hospitals. The German army recommended that twelve light hospitals, each able to accommodate two hundred sick or wounded men, accompany every corps of thirty thousand. The field hospitals followed the corps as it advanced and, as they filled with wounded, the army simply replaced them with new ones. To ensure success, the German Medical Department had acquired by 1870 full control of its men, transportation, and supplies.

Germany's ambulance equipment included stretchers carried by men; cacolets and litters borne by animals; country carts; ambulance carriages; wheeled supports for stretchers; and railway ambulance trains. Germany also devised a unique method for transforming the common Scotch haycart found in most European farmyards for ambulance transport. By improvising a suspensory apparatus similar in design to that used on the railroad, corpsmen were able to transport the wounded over rough terrain in conveyances that were surprisingly comfortable.[16]

The army also employed auxiliary aid societies and consulting civilian surgeons to assist ambulance detachments and field hospitals. Not only did field hospitals exhibit improved hygienic conditions through disinfectants and antiseptics but each soldier carried a "first field dressing." Although this was the first war to begin after the rise of so-called Listerism, antiseptic methods of wound management were still poorly

known and seldom practiced.[17] As a result of these improvements in
wound management, correspondent Archibald Forbes noted that the
German soldier went into battle reasonably prepared, carrying emergency bandages in his knapsack and an identification card around his neck.
Surgeons had only to dress wounds with the soldier's own medical
supplies and note on the card the severity of the wound, reducing the time
required for first aid and the work of physicians and surgeons who no
longer needed to duplicate a diagnosis.[18]

Although the French had been pioneers of the ambulance system,
French medical corps lacked command of their own organization until
1882. Unable to prepare adequately for and manage its support system,
the French were forced to delegate much of the responsibility to charity
and public-spirited voluntary nursing organizations. To make matters
worse, the French War Department had no organized system of railway
transport for its sick and wounded. Although the workshops at Montigny-
lès-Metz reconditioned a few railroad cars for ambulance transport, the
army moved most of its wounded on cars without stretchers or special
transport facilities. In contrast, the Bavarian army operated four complete
hospital trains, each consisting of twenty-nine cars, including seven
second- and third-class passenger cars available for those with minor
wounds; thirteen passenger cars fitted for recumbent patients; a car for
the surgeon and his assistants; a spare car for emergencies; a fuel car; six
freight cars, including one fitted as a kitchen; and storage cars. These
trains made thirty-nine trips during the war, transporting an estimated
ten thousand eight hundred patients.[19]

The German military tested various arrangements to support their
wounded in railway carriages. The Zavodovsky system (1873), named
after a Russian engineer, suspended litters from ropes fastened to hooks
on the sides of the carriages. This involved the use of field stretchers
furnished with mattresses and suspended by strong hemp girting, with
pads inserted between the stretcher and the side of the car to reduce
jolting. The hemp girting proved more satisfactory than the leather straps
and rubber rings used during the American Civil War that tended to split
or become too elastic.[20]

Grund's system converted railcars into ambulance wagons through the
use of semielliptical springs placed on the floor and used to support
stretchers. Similarly, the Count Beaufort system used a portable spring-
type mechanism to support the stretcher and reduce shaking. The Hamburg system employed a spring-suspender and clamp, which attached to
the roof of the carriage. Once connected, the mechanism supported a pair
of litters; with this innovation, sanitary personnel could make each

freight car accommodate ten to twelve patients. However, the system's designer, Hennicke, who exhibited his suspension system at the Vienna Universal Exposition of 1873, discovered that the roofs of many freight cars were too weak to support more than half the anticipated number of litters (plate 29).[21]

The importance of railways in removing the wounded was fully demonstrated in the Franco-Prussian War. "Every new development of railways," wrote Helmuth von Moltke (1800–1891), "is a military advantage; and for the national defense a few million on the completion of our railways is far more profitably employed than on our new fortresses." German efficiency distributed the wounded to various hospitals, moving the most serious cases to hospitals in towns nearest the front. Those recuperating from wounds transferred, by slow stages, from the battlefield to base hospitals. Although in theory the system eliminated the need for field hospitals, it presumed the maintenance of a regular railway communication, whether the army was on enemy soil or on home territory.[22]

By the end of the Franco-Prussian War, highly organized ambulance-train service had become a recognized part of the military organization of each of the major powers. In Germany it was known as *Lazarett-Zunge*, in France as *Train Sanitaire Permanent*, in Austria as *Sanität Zuge*, and in Italy as *Treno-Ospedale*. These permanent train services consisted of specially constructed rolling hospital cars, which served more seriously wounded and carried a specific complement of medical officers and support staff. They included kitchens, pharmacies, storerooms, and wards for the wounded. On average, these trains contained twenty-three cars, of which sixteen supported the wounded; the remainder were reserved for supplies and staff.[23]

Under ideal circumstances, sanitary personnel arranged support service, including the designation of appropriate accommodations, according to the evacuee's ability to bear the fatigue and discomfort of travel. In actual practice, however, the military found it more convenient to form hospital trains based on statistical averages, that is, eight passenger coaches for sitting patients, eight wagons for recumbent patients, and various baggage and support cars. As adopted by Austria, this composite train provided transport in proportions statistically predicted for the various classes of wounded.[24] In contrast, the Japanese perfected a system of evacuation that addressed the issue of statistical averaging by carefully timing the trains to leave at fixed hours each day. This practice created both a behavior and an expectation that boosted morale at the same time that it increased efficiency.[25]

In retrospect, the Franco-Prussian War served as a watershed for medical evacuation systems in the nineteenth century. It was the first major war to utilize the articles of the Geneva Convention and thereby to benefit from medical volunteers and large-scale support from neutrals. The war also tested the full capability of the railroad, the implications of small-arms technology and long-range weaponry, and the challenges they gave to existing stretcher-bearer systems. Although nations boasted impressive medical support and evacuation systems, including extensively organized zones for evacuating the wounded, they also recognized that modern weaponry had brought the effectiveness of these same systems into doubt. Planners had already predicted the awesomeness of concentrated firepower and the destructive capability that awaited the litter bearer in future wars. However, after a few years of anxiety and self-doubt, the war's aftermath left the public with a false sense of security as European powers scrambled to expand the boundaries of their influence.

Following the Franco-Prussian War, the German medical corps modified its hospital service by the *Kriegs Sanitäts Ordnung* of 1878 and the *Kriegs Etappen Ordnung* of 1887. As a result of these revisions, the German army's ambulance organization consisted of sanitary detachments, field hospitals, flying hospitals, hospital reserve depots, committees for the transport of the sick, and railway hospital trains. The administration of the ambulance service was in the hands of the chief of the ambulance sanitary staff. Next in command came the surgeons general of the armies in the field, the surgeons general of the army corps, and the surgeons in chief of the divisions and regiments. In addition, civil consulting surgeons and professors from the universities were attached to various military units and acted as advisors to the standing military surgical staff. The French ambulance system, as reorganized by the *Règlement* of 1884, was established on a structure closely resembling that of the German ambulance service.

France, Germany, Italy, and Russia made every effort to harmonize the organizational needs of their national societies and their respective armies. "In no future war," observed Furley, "will such freedom be allowed as was witnessed in 1870–71, and it is even doubtful if the services of neutrals from States, other than belligerents, will be allowed to intervene; or, if permitted to do so, they will have to serve under the orders of the army to which they may be attached."[26]

The French Red Cross Society reconstituted itself by dividing into three separate bodies, which governed themselves in peacetime but recognized the ultimate authority of the minister of war. Legislation in the 1880s determined the society's relationship to the military during war and directed its scope of activity in the distribution of support, assisting in transport, establishing hospitals, and, in general, affecting all medical service provided behind the war zone. In keeping with this legislation, the French Red Cross created thirty-nine depots for ambulance matériel that corresponded to the thirty-nine territorial divisions of the army. Annual maneuvers tested the readiness of personnel, and schools in Paris, Marseilles, Lille, and Nancy instructed support personnel. The French were determined to be prepared for the next war.[27]

Although the countries of western Europe instituted a series of adjustments in the 1870s as a result of the lessons learned from the Franco-Prussian War, other nations did not. Charles S. Ryan, an Australian surgeon with the Turkish army, recounted in *Under the Red Crescent* (1897) his experiences in several battles of the Russo-Turkish War (1877–78). Ryan explained how, after completing his medical work at Edinburgh, he traveled through Europe, eventually arriving at Plevna in July 1877. Enjoying the friendship of Osman Pasha, he agreed to become a military surgeon for the Ottoman army in the Red Crescent, the Turkish equivalent of the Red Cross. During the battle of Plevna, he noted the first of many mind-shattering experiences.

> As I looked up the Nicopolis Road I could see a long string of Bulgarian arabas, each drawn by two little white oxen, bringing the wounded down from the battlefield. Only the men who were gravely wounded were brought in these arabas, and hundreds had to drag themselves down on foot. As the rough, springless arabas jolted over the cobblestones of the Plevna street, the sufferings of the wounded men must have been excruciating. There was no field hospital to render first aid, and it is not easy to imagine the misery of an unfortunate wretch, say, with a compound fracture of the thigh, transported in a cart and without any surgical attendance from the field to the base hospital. . . . As far as the eye could reach stretched the long line of arabas, each with its load of suffering men. Every cart was driven by its Bulgarian owner, and escorted by a Turkish soldier to see that the Bulgarian did not dispatch the unhappy victims before their time.[28]

The *araba* (bullock cart), or ordinary country wagon, with its straw-covered floor and canopy raised overhead, transported most of the wounded during this war. It carried eight persons sitting or four reclining and, as it had no springs to relieve the jarring, promised little comfort to the wounded. As for the dead, medical attendants simply stacked them like cordwood on the wagon floor. "Sometimes," Ryan wrote, "when the carts came in I did not know which of the men were alive and which were dead, the living and the dead were lying so closely one on top of the other."[29]

England's Wars

The British were slow to change their customary ways of doing things. In engagements with the French in the early part of the nineteenth century, the British soldier had to wait for the fighting to end before receiving medical support. Not until the Crimean War did the British establish the Hospital Conveyance Corps, and this effort proved "so decided a failure" that the British transferred the responsibility for transporting wounded men to the Subsistence Department and its trains. Following the war, the British established the Medical Staff Corps, which also proved disappointing because of its dependence upon hired civilians.[30]

Both during and following the Crimean War, England initiated a series of actions designed to improve the health and welfare of the army. These efforts included two parliamentary committees (the Roebuck Committee and the Stafford Committee) to probe the organization and deficiencies of the Medical Department; the Royal Sanitary Commission, which studied the living conditions and health of the soldier; the Royal Warrant of October 1858, which set medical standards for military surgeons competitive with civilian practice; the maintenance of military statistics on the health of the army; the Indian army's Sanitary Commission, which brought improved health to troops in the Indian army; the Committee on Barrack Works and Hospital Construction, which remedied deficiencies in the hygiene of regimental hospitals; a code of regulations for the Purveyor's Branch, which had broken down completely during the Crimean War; and the opening of the Army Medical School at Fort Pitt (later moved to Netley) intended to train forty-five officers every six months on forms of emergency medicine not generally taught in civilian medical schools.[31] Most important was the formation of the Army Hospital Corps, established by Royal Warrant in 1857 and the successor to the ill-established Medical Staff Corps of 1855.

The Army Hospital Corps' two branches, the Purveyor's Branch and the Medical Branch, provided staff to the general and regimental hospitals. Although members of the corps wore the regimental uniform, they also wore a distinctive badge, carried no arms, and were assigned in times of war as litter bearers and in ambulance transport. In 1873, the inefficient regimental hospital system was discontinued and replaced with a new system of station and garrison hospitals. This more centralized approach eliminated much of the unnecessary duplication of equipment and services at the level of the regiment and promised better treatment for the sick and wounded. The Army Hospital Corps was reorganized, giving responsibility for medical stores and supplies to the medical officers, while the Supply and Transport Corps retained responsibility for buildings, water, fuel, and transport. Unfortunately, disciplinary control remained outside the responsibility of the Army Hospital Corps, and the unpopularity of these changes resulted in a shortage of new commissions.[32]

In 1876, the British army instituted new field-organization units that included bearer companies, movable field hospitals, stationary hospitals, general hospitals, sanitary detachments, medical stores, and hospital ships. This system provided medical support for the field-army organization of three divisions, a cavalry brigade, and corps troops. At the regimental level, each unit had a medical officer and sixteen stretcher-bearers.[33]

With the exception of the Crimean War, the British army fought all of its wars between 1815 and 1914 with non-European opponents—from sophisticated armies trained by Europeans to semiorganized troops, organized troops with primitive weapons, fanatics, guerrillas, and irregular cavalry. Peoples as diverse as the Sikhs, Kaffirs, Ashanti, Zulus, and Boers provided the grist for England's military experiences and the challenge of refining a consistent military and sanitary strategy. Because of their generally superior firepower, the British would fight rather than maneuver. "A rapid victory," wrote Hew Strachan in his *European Armies and the Conduct of War* (1983), "would prevent the dissolution of the regular army through sickness or lack of supplies. Moreover, if the opportunity to do battle was not taken, the enemy might disappear again, or his confidence might soon soar and the Europeans' moral superiority be lost."[34]

England's experiments with medical support units were thus determined in large part by its experiences in these wars, particularly in British India, where bearers typically were natives enlisted and organized into a bearer corps. These bearers, professional kahars who came chiefly from Oudh and Orissa, actually formed a distinct caste system, which had existed for more than a century. The bearers belonged to the regiments, as well as to the field hospitals. Using both dandies and dhoolies, they provided the basis for ambulance transport support to the British army.[35] Every field hospital carried with it twenty dhoolies, five with each section. There were 120 bearers, six to each dhoolie. In areas inhospitable to wheeled transport, the British relied upon the traditional camel litter, or kujjawa, and even experimented with a modified camel ambulance, invented by Lord Dundonald of the British army. The ambulance accommodated two recumbent or eight seated patients and proved so compact that, when disassembled, it could be carried on the back of a camel.[36]

During the South African campaign of 1899–1900, because of the small numbers of Royal Army Medical Corpsmen (R.A.M.C.) available, the British relied on the Indian army model, using a bearer company drawn from personnel of the field hospital. The bearers provided early treatment, supplied water and sedatives, and cairied the wounded on stretchers to collecting stations. From there, the wounded went in wagons to field hospitals. In addition, the British army relied upon civilian doctors, rank and file from the St. John Ambulance Brigade, the Volunteer Medical Staff Corps, and nursing sisters of the Army Nursing Reserve. The British Red Cross Society worked in close cooperation with the army to equip and operate hospital trains to move the sick and wounded. Private hospitals, equipped and sent out under the auspices of the Central Red Cross Council but administered by private committees, provided valuable service to the British army. The Portland Hospital, under the command of an officer of the R.A.M.C. appointed by the War Office, opened in January 1900 at Rondebosch. Attached to No. 3 General Hospital, the Portland Hospital consisted of four civilian sur-geons, six nurses, two noncommissioned officers of the R.A.M.C., and twenty-six men of the St. John Ambulance Brigade. Another private hospital, the Langman, supported one hundred beds and was situated on the line of communications at Bloemfontein. The Van Alen Hospital, the gift of an American, operated at Kimberley. Others included the Princess Christian Hospital; the Welsh Hospital, subscribed by the people of Wales; the Irish Hospital; the Scottish National Red Cross Hospital, organized by the St. Andrew Ambulance Association; and the Imperial Yeomanry Hospitals which, although supported by private monies, adopted a military-type organization.[37]

Ox wagons, hand transport, and other ambulance support vehicles suggested by Sir Thomas Longmore (1816–95) and George A. Otis (1781–1863) proved inadequate in the South African campaign because of the inability to secure trained animals; to make matters worse, most of the horses and mules imported for transport duties died of disease. Nevertheless, the country cart used to carry manure or fuel provided auxiliary transport in almost every war in the nineteenth century, and the Boer War was no exception. In South Africa, the military used ox trek wagons and Cape carts to move their sick and wounded. The trek wagon, eighteen to twenty feet long and four feet wide, carried two to four men lying down or twelve to sixteen sitting. Like most country wagons, it lacked springs, and straw mattresses and pillows provided the only available comfort. Both the wagons and the carts moved smoothly over grassy country but jolted over rocky terrain. The British also tested the

American wagonette, which was pulled by four to six mules and carried from six to eight sitting or two recumbent and four sitting men. The wagonette carried tent and cooking materials underneath its carriage which, during stops, could be set up to serve the wounded.[38] The British also employed a number of two-wheeled tongas, invented by Dhanjibhoy of Rawalpindi. Drawn by two mules, the tonga proved light, comfortable, and mobile and worked successfully with mounted troops. Another tonga, designed and built by a Colonel Jones, promised ready use in hill warfare and with mounted troops.[39]

For regular ambulance wagons, the British preferred a strong, light, easy-loading vehicle that would support four recumbent or twelve seated patients. Considering the advancements in weaponry, the British preferred that its ambulance wagons have a shape distinctive from all other army vehicles and a Red Cross emblem distinguishable at long range. Unfortunately, no wagon fulfilled all of these separate needs. The Mark III and Mark V ambulance wagons sacrificed comfort for strength in providing wheeled transport over extremely rough terrain. Able to carry only six patients, the Mark III was further hampered by braking difficulties and by the need to remove the backboard before loading recumbent patients. The Mark V had no compartments for carrying spare dressings, offered a poor turning radius and, like the Mark III, suffered from an inferior braking system. Other wagons used by the British in the Boer War included the New South Wales Army Medical Corps ambulance wagon (which closely resembled the Mark V) and a Gloucester wagon, later purchased by several private hospitals. Although the New South Wales wagon hung so low that it took on water when fording streams, it provided excellent accommodation for the wounded, whose field stretchers rested on two springs clamped to the floor of each compartment. The Gloucester wagon, used extensively in South Africa, was lighter and could be pulled by six mules. The floor of the wagon was three feet eight inches from the ground and was well fitted with lockers and tin water carriers.[40]

As a result of experiences in South Africa, England chose to rely on three ambulance wagons, recognizing that no single wagon could afford sufficient advantages to become the standardized model. The Mark I (Light), pulled by two horses and capable of transporting eight men sitting (or two lying and two sitting), remained the most popular wagon within the service. It required road space of twenty-three feet compared with forty to fifty feet needed by the heavier Mark V and Mark VI. The Mark I (Light) was easy to maneuver, used standard-sized and interchangeable parts (maximizing the use of partially damaged wagons), and proved practicable over rough terrain. In contrast, the heavier Mark V was pulled by four horses and carried fourteen sitting (or four lying and two sitting), while the Mark VI required six horses and carried fifteen sitting (or four lying and three sitting).[41]

CAVALRY

Between 1857 and 1870, cavalry shock tactics underwent profound changes, realizing too late in some cases the impact of increased firepower on cavalry organization and training. With rifled arms distinct from the smoothbore musketry of earlier wars, the cavalry came under fire eight hundred to a thousand yards from the enemy, allowing marksmen to counter their effectiveness at distant but deadly accurate ranges. Although still the chief means of mobility in the war theater, and continuing as a strategic element in reconnaissance, raids, and communication, the value of the cavalry had begun to decline.[42]

Notwithstanding the introduction of more deadly firepower and changes in war tactics, England continued to support thirty-one cavalry regiments along with its 114 battalions, even into the opening days of the Great War. The cavalry, divided into heavy, medium, and light, based on the size and weight of a horse and rider, were issued breech-loading carbines after the Crimean War and eventually the Martini-Henry (1878), Lee-Metford (1892), and Lee-Enfield (1901) rifles. By 1880, all cavalry carried a sword and carbine, while the lancers carried their own additional weapon.[43]

The British military in the late nineteenth century believed that the role of the mounted cavalry was about to be reborn. As one British observer noted: "We see a whole British army, largely owing to its insufficient mobility, checkmated at various points, and the situation cannot be altered until a large mounted force is sent to its relief."[44] The belief in a renaissance stemmed in large measure from minor colonial campaigns between 1870 and 1898 and from the rise of irregular cavalry, such as the Frontier Light Horse, the Mounted Rifles, and the Mounted Infantry. In effect, the cavalry retained an importance in England's colonial wars that had long been absent in European warfare. The shock effect of a cavalry charge in fighting the Sudanese, Samalis, and Sikhs no longer seemed as relevant in Europe. Despite the reality of the machine gun and the quickening developments in artillery firepower, the Kaffir War (1878) and operations against the Boers (1881) and in Egypt (1882) had given the cavalry an imagined importance far beyond its real effect in modern warfare. Ironically, at a time when the experience of war dictated other tactics, the British remained resolved to reintroduce the pre-Crimean era of the horse, lance, and saber. Indicative of this renewed attention was Frederick A. J. Bernhardi's book *Cavalry in Future Wars* (1906), Douglas Haig's *Cavalry Studies: Strategical and Tactical* (1907), and the publication of *Cavalry Journal*, begun in 1906 and taken over by the Cavalry School staff in 1908.[45]

Having committed itself to a total force of nearly twenty-two thousand regular and irregular cavalry, Britain's single most chronic problem became how best to support this mounted force with sufficient medical arrangements. Although European armies had developed elaborate schemes to clear the battlefield of their wounded, these plans fell conspicuously short in attending the needs of mounted troops. Cavalry out on patrol typically carried only bare essentials, which meant that no conveyances of any kind were available for those who became sick or wounded. When a soldier dropped from the ranks, he was carried on his own horse or that of a colleague until he reached camp. During cavalry movements, there was no rear zone for the mounted troops; the wounded simply accompanied their comrades until the assignment ended.

Because the cavalry supported the army in several ways (independent and strategic exploration, protective security, scouting, and intercommunication), arrangements for their wounded varied considerably. Many strategists objected to mixing mounted cavalry and wheeled vehicles because of the nature of their respective duties. It was only reasonable, they argued, for a mounted bearer division to accompany the cavalry. Nevertheless, the existing bearer companies of England's Army Hospital Corps were foot soldiers unable to keep pace with the cavalry. Major General Sir Herbert Stewart, recollecting his own experiences in Egypt, noted how "absolutely unsuitable" he found the support given by an unmounted bearer company for the cavalry division. In resolving this deficiency, Stewart ordered mounted bearers to accompany the cavalry. Later, in a memorandum to the Army Hospital Services Inquiry Committee in 1883, he unsuccessfully campaigned for the establishment of a permanent mounted bearer company.[46] A decade later, a Brigade Surgeon Williams, New South Wales Military Forces, organized a mounted bearer company to keep pace with the movements of cavalry in the field. Each bearer company consisted of five medical officers; eight noncommissioned officers; twenty-eight rank and file; ten light, two-horse ambulance wagons; two water carts; four storage wagons; and six horses to carry cacolets.[47]

Other forms of cavalry support included a saddle fixture (plate 30) designed by Colonel H. G. Hathaway, R.A.M.C., that prevented a wounded soldier, even an unconscious one, from falling from his saddle. A semicir-

cle of light metal, padded on the inside and covered in leather, provided
the support. The British also experimented with bicycles improvised to
support a stretcher and used to transport wounded cavalry to collection
areas accessible to wagons. Later, the military considered using privately
owned motorcars requisitioned to accommodate the wounded.[48]

Aside from these innovations, the British Royal Army Medical Corps
continued to debate the most appropriate type of ambulance evacuation
system for its mounted troops. For all its good intentions, ambulance
transport for mounted cavalry remained essentially the same as for
infantry; moreover, as the war in South Africa had demonstrated, Britain's
ambulance evacuation units were ill equipped to assist troops split into
small fighting groups.[49]

AMERICAN RETRENCHMENT

Except for a short-term force in Texas to persuade France to withdraw
from Mexico, Union military forces rapidly demobilized following the
Civil War. By the end of Reconstruction, the army had reduced in
numbers to 27,442 troops, while the U.S. Navy retained only fifty-two of
its nearly seven hundred ships. The American army was thus one-seventh
the size of Britain's and a twentieth of France's. With the American
continent safe from monarchy and the nation focusing its energies on
territorial and economic expansion, the army skirmished with the Indians
between 1866 and 1890 and assisted states in protecting private property
during strikes and general labor unrest. Until the revival of the National
Guard, the army was little more than a national police force empowered
to quell social disturbances.[50]

Grant's strategy of destroying the South's will to fight applied as well in
the postwar era for the American Indian. While the United States had
attempted—albeit inconsistently—to accommodate both the needs of the
Indian nations and the desires of white settlers in the early years of the
American republic, the passage of the Homestead Act of 1862 opened a
new chapter in misunderstandings, deceit, and armed clashes between
Indians and homesteaders. With these clashes emerged a federal policy of
repression, which included the advance of the railroads over disputed
land, the destruction of the buffalo herds, and the forced migration of
broken tribes and once-proud warriors onto reservations.[51]

The resurgence in the 1880s of Manifest Destiny under the banner of
social Darwinism, Christianity, and the white man's burden resulted in an
effort to modernize the armed forces. Technology and imperialism joined
hands to build lighter and stronger guns, iron hulls and armor, better
engines and increased speed, and breech-loading rifles with longer ranges

and greater velocity. Both the army and the navy called for the refurbishment of coastal defenses. The Endicott Board of 1886, under the chairmanship of Secretary of War William C. Endicott, recommended the rehabilitation of coastal fortifications, including a major investment in breech-loading rifles, mortars, machine guns, electric searchlights, floating batteries, and mines. In 1888, Congress created the Army Board of Ordnance and Fortifications, which resulted in a mixed system of government-owned plants (Watervliet Arsenal and Washington Naval Yard) and private-sector suppliers (Carnegie and Bethlehem).[52]

General William T. Sherman, Rear Admiral Steven B. Luce, and their protégés Emory Upton, Arthur L. Wagner, and Alfred Thayer Mahan profoundly influenced military and strategic thinking in the latter decades of the nineteenth century and in the early twentieth century. Seeking to encourage the advancement of a professional officer corps, Sherman advocated postgraduate military education (e.g., at the Engineering School of Applications at Willett's Point, New York; and at the School of Application for Infantry and Cavalry at Fort Leavenworth, Kansas) beyond the military academy, and he called for the publication of professional military journals. Upton's admiration for the German military system was reflected in his books—*The Armies of Asia and Europe* (1878), *A New System of Infantry Tactics* (1873), and *The Military Policy of the United States* (1904)—which gave new insight into military readiness and professional competence. Equally important were the writings of Lieutenant Wagner, who was sent to Leavenworth as an instructor of military art. His *Campaign of Königgrätz* (1889), *Service of Security and Information* (1893), and *Organization and Tactics* (1895) became the standard authorities for many years. Luce was responsible for the establishment of the War Naval College at Newport, Rhode Island, in 1884 and urged naval officers to develop "scientific" strategies and principles for sea warfare comparable to the classic treatises of land warfare. The genius of Mahan, who taught at the Naval War College, provided the impressive trilogy *The Influence of Sea Power upon History, 1660–1783* (1890); *The Influence of Sea Power upon the French Revolution and Empire, 1793–1812* (1892); and *Sea Power in Its Relations to the War of 1812* (1905), a trilogy that set forth a philosophy that would influence nations worldwide. While reformers in the army sought to break the mold of a civilian-controlled and uniformly weak force of twenty-eight thousand officers and men, the navy entered the twentieth century as an ascending world sea power.[53]

Unfortunately, many of the benefits affecting medical evacuation were lost in the post–Civil War period. "The whole military establishment fell back almost to its ante-bellum status," complained Major Charles Smart in 1893, with medical officers seldom able to obtain either men or matériel suitable for hospital support. "The commanding officer disliked to lose good soldiers from the ranks," Smart observed, "but readily spared any man who was broken down, valueless from innate stupidity, or worse than worthless from dissipation." After laboring to build a hospital system, the most energetic medical officer found himself "subsided into a state of resignation" as a result of misplaced priorities. According to Smart,

> The men whom he could get, not the men whom he wanted, were those that the medical officer had to prepare for the duties of giving first aid to the injured; and afterward, when, by dint of care and assiduous personal attention to their physical and moral well-being he had repaired the broken constitution, awakened the intelligence, uprooted the evil habits, and endowed these men with possibilities of future worth, they were probably transferred to the ranks and the hospital provided with substitutes as worthless as those that had originally been sent.[54]

In March 1887, Congress authorized the establishment of the Hospital Corps, a special unit under the direction of the Army Medical Department. This act removed one of the great obstacles in the way of first aid by directing medical officers to select, educate, drill, and discipline members of the Hospital Corps. With this authorization, according to Smart, "officers began earnestly to build up the organization and so systematize its work that the same principles would regulate its action in times of peace as in times of stupendous war."[55] The Hospital Corps, as revised March 16, 1896, was comprised of enlisted men performing services in garrison, camp, and field (including ambulance service), who were permanently attached to the Army Medical Department and not counted as part of the effective strength of the army. The law mandated examinations before a board of medical officers for all hospital stewards and the enlistment of privates as wardmasters, cooks, nurses, and attendants in hospitals and as stretcher-bearers and ambulance attendants in the field.[56]

Most importantly, the Hospital Corps organization ensured first aid to the fighting soldier during battle and eliminated the need for men to drop out of the line to help a wounded comrade to the rear. This depletion of the ranks, which had so infuriated commanders in the field, was no longer justified or necessary. Still, however, the U.S. Army *Regulations* provided for the education in first aid of four men from each company whose duty outside soldiery included assisting the wounded from the field until relieved by members of the Hospital Corps.[57]

The Spanish-American War

Notwithstanding the appeals and efforts of medical officers, the American military gave little thought to ambulance support in the late nineteenth century, and when the nation went to war against Spain in April 1898, its medical evacuation system had not visibly improved in the thirty-three years since the Civil War. The United States entered the war with insufficient equipment and training and was inexperienced in handling or supplying large numbers of troops. The United States had no organized, equipped, and trained ambulance company or field hospital; it relied instead upon improvised support with many unintended consequences. So mishandled were the medical supplies for the Cuban expedition that, without the support of the Red Cross, the Medical Department would have been unable to attend the needs of the army. Medical supplies were lost in freight yards and remained undiscovered for weeks. One reason for these poor conditions was the army's view that the Medical Department, as a noncombatant branch, contributed little to the general mission of the military; serving an ancillary role, it ranked secondary to other more important needs.[58]

With the outbreak of war, Congress authorized the appointment of a chief surgeon to the staff of each corps, division, or brigade; and the president allocated a surgeon and two assistant surgeons for each regiment of volunteer infantry, engineers, and cavalry. In addition, Surgeon General George M. Sternberg, a research scientist in bacteriology and epidemiology, was authorized to hire additional assistant surgeons on contract. Sternberg employed some six hundred fifty contract assistant surgeons. Unfortunately, few of these physicians understood military discipline or had any appreciation for the army's sanitation needs in the field. Most were political appointments beyond the purview of the surgeon general, as were many of the seventeen thousand contract nurses employed by the Medical Department.[59]

To complicate matters, Sternberg and Colonel Charles R. Greenleaf, chief surgeon of the Fifth Army Corps, found themselves in the unenviable situation of having to provide medical supplies and equipment that they had been prevented from stockpiling earlier. Few regiments had medical equipment of any kind; and, despite Sternberg's appeal to governors to ensure that their troops were given ample medical supplies, sixteen states sent no medical matériel with their troops. Moreover, Sternberg could not order the Quartermaster's Department to give priority shipping to needed medical supplies. The Quartermaster's Department refused to pack Medical Department matériel together; instead, it parceled out medical matériel among freight allotments, requiring time-consuming sorting of shipments when they arrived at port. Equipment for a two-hundred-bed hospital remained lost for weeks on a rail siding.[60]

The outbreak of typhus in the camps caused Sternberg to abolish the regimental hospital system and to replace it with the larger divisional and general hospital unit. However, staffing the larger units remained a problem because Congress and many state governors chose to retain the regimental unit. Sternberg also fitted three hospital ships, one of which was a refitted cattle boat, while another had only a brief career: it sank in stormy weather during a coaling operation.[61]

Despite the Army Medical Department's aversion to assistance from voluntary and charitable organizations, it was unable to provide proper care for the sick and wounded and gave grudging acquiescence to their efforts. The American Red Cross Society established supply depots in all the large camps, dispensing ice, medicines, dressings, and hospital supplies. Following the surrender of Santiago, the Red Cross vessel *State of Texas* under the command of Clara Barton (1821–1912) became the first ship to enter the harbor on an errand of mercy. After the war ended, Barton and her staff sailed for Havana to deliver aid to the *reconcentrados* in the besieged city.

The American Red Cross, with the approval of the United States government, sent to Cuba six ambulances purchased from the Studebaker Brothers Manufacturing Company of South Bend, Indiana. The ambulances were of the same design as the Tooker ambulance, formerly built by Studebaker for the government, and similar in design and construction to the ordinary delivery wagons made by Studebaker. Painted Prussian blue and chrome yellow, the ambulances carried four stretchers, with the bottom two stretchers hinged to move aside to accommodate sitting patients or personnel.[62] Stephen E. Barton, a nephew of Clara Barton and chairman of the President's Committee for Cuban Relief (later known as the Central Cuban Relief Committee), shipped the six ambulances to Havana aboard the *Port Victor* in July 1898. After a forty-seven-day delay following their arrival in Havana, the military reloaded the ambulances on the schooner *Mary E. Morse* bound for Baracoa and Gibara on the northern coast of Santiago province. Arriving on September 22, the ambulances again met with delays in unloading and had not been put into use by the time of the armistice on October 24. In disgust, Stephen Barton ordered the ambulances returned to New York. In Puerto Rico, however, two Studebaker ambulances provided valuable support for soldiers and supplies. Unfortunately, as Clara Barton noted, the ambulance wagons became a "delicate responsibility, as everybody seemed to regard them as free pleasure coaches in which the Red Cross was eager to take the town to ride."[63]

Newspaper reports, along with congressional concern and complaints from surgeons attached to volunteer units from the States and from men like Theodore Roosevelt, led to demands for an inquiry into the operation of the Medical Department and the competence of the surgeon general. Although some rose to Sternberg's defense, a furor arose over his leadership and the bunglings reported during the Santiago campaign. However, an internal investigation carried out by Major Victor C. Vaughan, Major Walter Reed, and Major Edward O. Shakespeare contained no criticism of Sternberg's administration of the Medical Department. The Dodge Commission, appointed by President William McKinley to investigate the conduct of the war and headed by General Grenville M. Dodge, concluded in its report in 1900 that the Medical Department's lack of preparedness had been due to factors over which it had little or no control. It blamed Congress for reducing the numbers of assistant surgeons, failing to authorize a volunteer hospital corps, and refusing to authorize sufficient appropriations for medical supplies and equipment. The report also criticized the Quartermaster's Department for its decision to ship supplies by freight in order to save money, for the unsatisfactory method with which it loaded and unloaded medical stores at points of debarkation, and for its outright failure to deliver supplies when needed. The commission found that, of forty fully equipped ambulances intended for General William R. Shafter's Fifth Corps, the general had directed thirty-seven to be left behind. Reminiscent of the British Crimean Expeditionary Force, the Fifth Army Corps was forced to rely upon mule-drawn army wagons as ambulances, which proved wholly inadequate because of road conditions.[64]

The *Dodge Report* also criticized the politically appointed medical officers of regiments. According to the commission's findings, many had little understanding of camp sanitation and, not being knowledgeable about military training and authority, were ill prepared to enforce sanitary regulations that would have minimized infectious diseases. In an earlier speech, presented before the American Medical Association (A.M.A.) in Columbus, Ohio, in 1899, Sternberg provided an analysis that was strikingly similar to that later made by the Dodge Commission.

> The medical officers of regiments . . . were competent professionally, but they were called upon to assume new responsibilities for which they had no special training. Unfortunately, hygiene and practical sanitation are subjects which receive little attention in our medical schools or from physicians and

surgeons engaged in the practice of medicine. But even in those cases in which the regimental surgeon was fully aware of the importance of camp sanitation and urgent in his sanitary recommendations, he was unable to control the sanitary situation unless the regimental and company officers enforced the necessary measures for protecting the health of the command. And just here is the fundamental difficulty when we are dealing with new levies of troops. The officers and enlisted men of our volunteer regiments were as a rule intelligent, patriotic and brave, but they were not disciplined. . . . And in the absence of discipline it is impracticable to enforce proper sanitary regulations in camp. The surgeon-general may formulate sanitary regulations, and the general commanding an army corps or a division may issue the necessary orders, but in the absence of discipline these orders will not be enforced.[65]

THE PHILIPPINES INSURRECTION

In the seven-hour battle of Manila Bay (May 1, 1898), Commodore George Dewey's U.S. Navy Asiatic Squadron destroyed the Spanish fleet of cruisers and gunboats, making the United States Navy supreme in the archipelago's waters. Since the capital city of Manila remained in Spanish hands, however, Dewey imposed a blockade and requested that a small U.S. Army force occupy the capital as a means of forcing Spain to accept peace in Cuba. General Wesley Merrit arrived in the Philippines on July 25 and, joining forces with Filipino nationalists under the command of General Emilio Aguinaldo, occupied Manila on August 13. The next day, Merrit received the Spanish capitulation and proclaimed military occupation of the Philippines.

Merrit's capture of Manila marked the end of active hostilities in the Spanish-American War and the beginning of a breakdown in relations between the United States government and Aguinaldo's nationalists who, having established a provisional government in June 1898 and having proclaimed independence from Spain, had supported the American troops in Manila on the assumption that the United States would grant freedom and independence to the islands. When Aguinaldo learned of the Treaty of Paris (December 10, 1898) and of the Spanish cession of the Philippines to the United States for twenty million dollars, he led the Filipinos in armed revolt against U.S. rule.

Despite broken promises and Aguinaldo's hopes for independence, President McKinley intended for the Filipinos to learn the "benefits" of American government. In other words, American designs included a colonial government in the Philippines. The United States was determined to exercise its sovereignty in the region, and the Filipinos were equally resolved to be independent. The results of this standoff tested the tenacity of both defender and pacifier. Few Americans realized at the time, however, that the archipelago consisted of more than seven thousand islands, with a total area of 115,026 square miles, five major linguistic groups, and a climate and terrain that could "be greater adversaries than any human enemy."[66]

The war in the Philippines divided into two parts: one of preparation, siege, and occupation of Manila; the other embracing a succession of fierce battles and severe marches on Malolos, Calumpit, and San Fernando. With only an initial twenty-six thousand troops present in the Philippines, the United States could barely establish a presence except in the provincial capitals and in key cities. Thus, to suppress the uprising, the United States employed an augmented force of seventy thousand men against a Filipino army almost as large. The army's three-pronged offensive against Aguinaldo's army on the Luzon Plains resulted in the withdrawal of the Filipino army into the mountainous region of northern Luzon, where it conducted a guerrilla-type war to counteract the larger and more conventionally organized American units. Aguinaldo abandoned all pretense to conventional battle tactics and transformed his remaining forces into guerrilla bands that relied on skirmishes, raids, and ambushes. Americans learned quickly that guerrilla warfare in jungle settings abrogated both the rules of traditional engagement and the means of supporting and evacuating the wounded.

Although ambulance companies had been organized for the northern campaign, consisting originally of six ambulances, a number of carabao carts, litters, and hospital personnel, the nature of the terrain convinced the Hospital Corps to disband the companies and assign them elsewhere.[67] In this environment, the ambulance wagons sent from the United States were too heavy for the soft, muddy roads. In fact, the mountainous trails proved too tough and the turns too short for even the travois. A one-horse litter, with the horse hitched between the front ends of bamboo poles and two men carrying the rear ends, was sometimes used in the foothills to bring in the wounded. This improvisation seemed to work, but it could not be used in much of the countryside owing to thick vegetation.[68] There, corpsmen improvised litters from materials found on the trails and sought additional help from prisoners, who were either hired or impressed into service, and from Chinese coolies.[69]

Because the Chinese inhabitants of the islands had been poorly treated by the nationalists, many chose to collaborate with the Americans, acting as guides, spies, and litter bearers for the sick and wounded.[70] One member of the Hospital Corps and two "Chinos" constituted a litter squad. These, with whatever medical officers and acting stewards might join the expedition, would work at the firing line, administer first aid, and remove the wounded to a convenient dressing station in the rear, from whence they could be evacuated by ambulance, bull cart, or such transportation as the country afforded, to the nearest permanent station.[71] The conventional first-aid station on the field, with an ambulance station and a brigade hospital in the rear of battle, simply did not work in the "running fights" that the troops experienced when facing guerrilla fighters. Instead, the wounded were dressed where they fell, and permanent dressings were applied in a town or settlement after it had been taken.[72]

When the advance reached San Fernando, the corps built a stationary hospital to accommodate men exhausted or wounded in pursuit of the enemy. Later, as troops moved in small commands after the insurgent Filipinos, small field hospitals were set up to accompany the expeditionary forces; from these jungle environments, the wounded were evacuated to coastal hospitals in litters made from bamboo and strips of bark, native carts, handcarts, boxcars equipped with cots, and eventually hospital trains. The railroad became an important artery of communication for men and supplies as well as important in the evacuation of sick and wounded men. To facilitate the handling of the sick and wounded, two railroad cars were fitted with cots, water closets, ice chests, medicines, and cooking apparatus. The trip from the end of the line to Manila took approximately twenty-four hours.[73]

Considering the difficult transportation and the need to move the wounded by various extemporaneous means, medical corpsmen lamented their ability to provide suitable dressings. Wound dressings, no matter how skillfully applied, "were wrenched loose by the fearful jolting and switching of those most abominable vehicles over the . . . roads," wrote Lieutenant Colonel A. A. Woodhull. "I seriously contemplated at one time dismissing the carts and having the wounded carried by hand, but I found the road was so full of pitfalls and boulders that litter bearers were unable to keep their feet and would certainly have dropped their burdens."[74]

Because of the long line of communication from the forward troops to the southern seacoast, "post hospitals arose as rapidly as the smoke from the camp fire," providing support for the sick and wounded, with the troops garrisoning the points held as the army proceeded.[75] By December 1900, the Hospital Corps had established nearly four hundred lightly equipped field hospitals along the lines of communication and had positioned them to take advantage of rail transportation to Manila.[76] Each isolated post required the services of a physician with supplies and equipment. This requirement was a severe challenge to the Medical

Department, now called upon to provide a ratio of physicians to soldiers far in excess of any previous experience. At any one time, the dressing stations or light field hospitals cared for as many as 14 percent of the sick and wounded.[77] Many of the stations were from four to ten miles apart and without medical officers, leaving the Hospital Corps to perform its medical duties as best it could; and many medical officers were "obliged to attend from three to five stations, visiting them at great personal risk, since the country [was] invested with ladrones and insurgents, and it [was] not always possible to obtain proper escort." To assist in supply, the regular Hospital Corps in the Philippines supplemented its numbers with several hundred civil contract surgeons, many of whom had little experience with military medicine. Moreover, when the term of service of these contract doctors expired, many demanded to be sent home. As a result, as many as 120 posts operated without surgeons.[78]

The seriously ill were sent from these small makeshift hospitals to regimental hospitals or to hospitals placed further back along the lines of communication. The base hospitals, usually converted buildings of a public character, were fully equipped and had an average capacity of about fifty beds. These hospitals were in close touch with Manila, which maintained large general hospitals with up to a thousand beds for those requiring special treatment. From there, soldiers transferred to general hospitals in San Francisco, California. The percentage of deaths among the wounded was 6.9 percent; the percentage of those killed outright was 8 percent; and the percentage of deaths to all casualties was 14.96 percent. Medical men attributed the favorable outcome of most wounds to the use of first-aid packets and the promptness with which aseptic treatment was applied.[79]

4
Old and New Thinking

Although strategists at the turn of the century predicted that armies would fight future wars with weapons too destructive to allow immediate relief for the wounded, most medical planners were unable to suggest support and evacuation systems other than aid "at the first practicable moment." Generally, military planners recognized that larger fighting forces would become embroiled in future wars; that wounded might lie unattended during a battle; and that, in order to save lives, assistance would require haste and efficiency when the fighting ended. Nevertheless, few planners considered meeting these emergencies with anything but more conveyances and additional volunteers. They willingly experimented with new techniques, but not until the development of the motorized ambulance did armies finally discover an effective alternative to the prevailing medical evacuation system.[1]

LITTERS AND OTHER SUPPORT

During the last decades of the nineteenth century, military attention focused on options for rapid removal of the wounded from battle, including light, wheeled vehicles drawn by hand, bicycles designed to carry a loaded litter, and wheelbarrows. At the Centennial Exposition of 1876, participating governments displayed a wide array of ambulance vehicles, stretchers, and small handcars. The Medical Department of the U.S. Army exhibited hand litters, ambulance wagons, railroad cars fitted with extra springs and supports for stretchers, and models of ships fitted for transporting the wounded. The U.S. Navy also introduced an ambulance cot that would allow patients to be passed through small hatchways or narrow stairways and would serve as an invalid's chair when necessary.[2]

In 1883 and 1884, military planners in Vienna, Paris, Aldershot, and Geneva experimented with a portable electric-light wagon designed to assist stretcher-bearers in seeking, identifying, and evacuating wounded. At Gratz, men in the Austrian medical service carried portable electric, battery-fed lanterns in their knapsacks. During the Boer War, the British used acetylene searchlights to find the wounded at night; and at Port Arthur, the Russians experimented with flares suspended from balloons for the same purpose.[3]

The French army in 1893 authorized a one-horse cart carrying stretchers to accompany each battalion of one thousand soldiers as it went into battle. This meant bringing wagon transportation directly into the area of the greatest number of casualties and supplementing stretcher-bearers with additional supplies. Other nations, including the Japanese in China in 1894 and 1895, employed packhorses to carry stretchers into the battle areas. In still other situations, bearers carried extra litters as they marched at the rear of the regiment.[4]

At the Fifth International Conference at Rome in April 1892, the king and queen of Italy announced a competition for the best conveyance for removing the wounded from a battlefield. An innovation that followed in the wake of this and similar requests was the bicycle ambulance (plate 31), developed to minimize the work of the stretcher-bearer. The Austrian medical corps, for example, devised a bicycle that, when disassembled, served as a two-wheeled litter. Another variation was the "cycle ambulance," manufactured by the Remington Arms Company and constructed from two tandem bicycles connected by tubing. Riders occupied the back seats of the tandems while the front seats and pedals were removed to support a detachable litter.[5]

From time to time, the military experimented with variations of the wheelbarrow. American painter, illustrator, and sculptor Frederic Remington (1861–1909), a special correspondent for *Harper's Weekly* during the Geronimo campaign in the West, devised what he called a *litter-carrier*. His invention consisted of a regulation litter that fastened to a carrier by a removable pin; the frame, with three-leaved springs, had a single rubber-rim wheel two feet in diameter. With two bearers, one pulling and one pushing, the litter-carrier transported wounded over long distances without tiring the bearers. Unfortunately, Remington's invention proved awkward over rough and broken terrain and dangerous during a firefight because it exposed both patient and bearers.[6]

Despite efforts to introduce new medical transport, the hand litter or stretcher remained the principal conveyance for medical evacuation. Litters came in two basic forms: those with fixed handles and those that telescoped for use in ambulance wagons. Through the 1890s, the American military relied on both forms until it discontinued the latter to encourage greater uniformity. The regulation American litter of the 1890s consisted of a canvas bed measuring six feet long and twenty-two inches wide, supported by two poles measuring seven and one-half feet, and two jointed braces or traverses. The litter had four-inch legs designed to raise the patient off the ground; the legs curved into a loop or stirrup, which improved stability and made the litter easy to slide along the floor of the ambulance wagon. The German litter had an iron strap that served a similar purpose, while the English litter came with a wooden roller to facilitate ambulance loading.[7]

Nations differed on their use of a litter pillow. The French litter, for example, offered a raised canvas headrest, while the German litter provided a separate and adjustable headrest. The English litter, on the other hand, contained a horsehair pillow that was available only during ambulance transport. In contrast, the American litter provided neither pillow nor headrest; when necessary, attendants simply improvised with a coat or a blanket. The American litter weighed twenty-four pounds with shoulder slings, the French weighed twenty-five, and the English, thirty-two pounds.[8]

Messrs. Fischer and Company of Heidelberg were principal manufacturers of ambulance equipment in the late nineteenth century, marketing their wares across Europe and America through printed catalogs containing photographs and drawings of transport and surgical appliances. They included in their catalog the Pirogoff high-wheeled hand litter, Gablenz's hand litter on two lower wheels, chair litters, and cacolets. These and other conveyances promised both portability and durability. The popularity of light, portable equipment stemmed in part from Europe's sprawling overseas empires. Governments desired collapsible litters and other ambulance equipment that would pack for easy transport abroad (plates 32, 33).

In countries or territories with large populations, stretcher-bearers drawn from the local civilian population remained the most practical and efficient means of medical evacuation. During the battle of Sha-ho on

October 12, 1904, the Japanese relied upon Chinese carts and coolie labor for almost all stretcher transport between the dressing stations and the field hospitals. During the Philippine insurrection in 1899, the United States Army allotted twelve Chinese coolies to each regiment as litter bearers. This method also proved successful in 1899–1900 in Natal, where the British pressed into service a bearer corps of twelve hundred European refugees from the Transvaal and eight hundred Indian coolies. The army relied on this improvised bearer corps for transferring patients from field hospitals to railway trains after Colenso, Spion Kop, and other actions near Pieter's Hill.[9]

AMBULANCE PROCEDURES

Ambulance procedures did not vary much from one country to another. The litter bearers worked in squads of four, known individually as Numbers l, 2, 3, and 4. Numbers 2 and 3 carried the litter, while numbers 1 and 4 walked on either side. Number 1 acted as squad leader. Each carried water and field dressings, but number 4 also carried a pouch containing field surgical supplies. When operating in an exposed field with wounded men, numbers 1 and 4 determined a wounded soldier's condition. This evaluation involved an understanding of those conditions that affected the soldier's transportation (i.e., whether shock, hemorrhage, or fractures required attention; whether the soldier could have water, with or without a stimulant; and whether he might faint or have difficulty breathing).[10]

The litter or bearer squad in the 1890s carried pouches containing a candle and matches; two field tourniquets; aromatic spirits of ammonia for treating internal hemorrhage and shock; scissors; dressing forceps; a jackknife; pins, needles, and thread; antiseptic bandages; adhesive plaster; petroleum jelly; a hard-rubber iodoform sprinkler; two sponges; a first-aid package; sublimated lint and boric wool; and wire splints with tapes and buckles. The first-aid package contained a strong rubber cloth, nine inches square, and two yards of sublimated gauze and cambric, a triangular bandage, and safety pins.[11] With these materials, litter bearers attempted to arrest hemorrhage, remove foreign bodies from the wound, prevent bacterial invasion, and protect the patient from injury during transportation by opening the wound and removing the dried or clotted blood and other foreign matter. The litter bearers then checked hemorrhage, cleared the wound, dried it with antiseptic gauze, dusted it with iodoform, and covered the area with gauze and a bandage. In cases of fracture, bearers applied splints, improvising when necessary with rifles, sword blades, or other temporary supports.[12]

The value of the first-aid dressing applied on the battlefield by the wounded soldier, a comrade, or a corpsman was not universally acknowledged. Although first-aid dressings were used by the British as early as the Crimean War, these dressings consisted merely of a calico bandage and four pins intended to prevent gross soiling of a wound. Not until the Sudan campaign of 1894 did the British dressing have some antiseptic utility, being made of two pads of carbolized cloth, a gauze bandage, pins, and a triangular bandage—all sealed in tinfoil and covered by parchment. The French military surgeons Venant A. L. Legouest and Edmund Delorme did not favor its use and, until 1889, no such packages were distributed to the French army. In 1892, the United States officially adopted first-aid packages for front-line dressings. By 1896, each officer and enlisted man included one of these packages in his equipment. During the Spanish-American War, the surgeon general issued 270,000 first-aid packages to the troops in Cuba and Puerto Rico. The package contained two antiseptic compresses of sublimated gauze in oiled paper; one antiseptic sublimated cambric bandage, with safety pin; and one triangular Esmarch bandage, with safety pin. However, the package proved too bulky for the soldier to carry; instead, doctors in field hospitals used the dressings.[13]

Following this "initial relief," the stretcher detachment carried the soldier to a collecting or dressing station close to the fighting line but in an area of relative safety, usually under some shelter. There, noncommissioned officers and men attended minor wounds, while the medical officer treated the more serious cases. The medical officer's supplies included the Esmarch tourniquet; chloroform; a hypodermic syringe with morphine tablets; and vials containing tablet doses of acetanilide, sulfate of quinine, compound cathartic pills, corrosive sublimate, and sal ammoniac. Over his shoulder he carried a field case containing scalpel, amputating knife, saw, scissors, forceps, Nelaton's probe, needles, silk and wire ligature, and catheter.[14]

At the dressing station, the duties of the surgeon included averting life-threatening dangers, such as hemorrhage or shock, substituting the ligature for the tourniquet, extracting bullets or fragments of shell, securing fractured bones, and tagging those men requiring prompt attention at the field hospital. The medical officer maintained a book of tags on which he detailed information to hospital surgeons for each case. The tags fastened over a button on the patient's chest. Ambulance wagons then transported the wounded to a field hospital.[15]

From an organizational point of view, the medical evacuation systems represented three distinct zones: collecting, evacuating, and distributing.

The collecting zone was the area of active operations; the evacuating zone, one of lines of communication; and the distributing zone, the base and home territory. In practice, the three zones tended to overlap. The collecting zone included the regimental units, field ambulances, and the cavalry field ambulances. The evacuating zone included the clearing hospitals and ambulance trains; while the distributing zone involved the stationary hospitals, general hospitals, hospital ships, and military hospitals at home. In England, linkage among the zones came under the responsibility of the director of medical and sanitary services at army headquarters.[16]

Factors affecting evacuation included the nature of the wounds, the number of wounded, the character of the battle, the physical condition of the troops, and the types and quantities of medical support. Additional elements concerned the number of available ambulance stations, the nature of the terrain, the availability of transportation, the meteorological conditions; and whether troops had proper first-aid packages, whether there was access to civilian labor, and whether physicians used diagnosis tags.[17]

For medical planners, the clearing or field hospital, which temporarily received and cared for the wounded prior to evacuation, became the pivotal point in their collection and distribution. It was the direct link between all three zones and the unit for channeling the flow of wounded between divisional ambulances and railways. Clearing hospitals existed for each division, and their position at the head of each line of communication determined in large part the efficiency and effectiveness of medical care. Without an efficient system of evacuation, the chances of clogging operations with casualties became all too real.

Every clearing hospital tried not to become too far removed from the forward lines of the division. In South Africa, for example, the British placed their field hospitals so far behind the division that the lines of communication became tenuous at best. As a result, the British found it necessary to subdivide the clearing hospital in an effort to bridge the distance between the field ambulances and the railheads. When this occurred, the clearing hospital formed "a series of intermediate posts for the temporary care of sick and wounded passing down the line."[18]

BEGINNINGS OF DOUBT

At the same time that manufacturers designed and produced ambulance equipment for Europe's armies, sanitary personnel and military strategists were beginning to question the very premises of their medical evacuation systems. Their questioning was based on several factors: the

changing character of wounds produced by modern weapons, the improvements in field surgery, the extended fronts and open formations of
modern warfare, and the increased depth of the zone of fire. While in
earlier wars the number killed had equaled or exceeded the number of
wounded, modern surgical science had greatly reduced mortality among
the wounded, a situation that forced armies to increase significantly those
units supporting the collection, evacuation, and distribution of wounded.

One principal reason behind this new thinking was the innovations in
small-bore rifles with increased velocity and effectiveness at long distances. Developments in weapons technology, in metallurgy, ballistics,
and precision engineering had made possible the replacement of smoothbore muskets and muzzle-loaders with rifles accurate to five hundred
yards and artillery effective at ranges of more than two thousand yards.
The impact of improved small arms, long-range artillery, and quick-firing
machine guns increased the destructive potential of war. The consequences of this technology on the battlefield, particularly upon the
traditional battalion columns, was nothing short of revolutionary.[19]

The British, French, and Austrians continued to employ muzzle-
loading rifles in their 1854 and 1859 campaigns, but the Prussians had
moved to the breech-loading Dreyse needle-fire rifle (so called because
the cartridge was ignited by a steel pin driven into the base by the
hammer) as early as 1843. The Seven Weeks' War of 1866 saw the first
European demonstration of breech-loading weapons. At the battle of
Königgrätz, the Austrian army, armed with the older, muzzle-loading,
rifled artillery that fired case loads or shrapnel, was confronted by
Prussians armed with breech-loading rifled cannon and breech-loading
needle-guns, sighted to four hundred yards. With the Prussian infantry
firing six shots to the Austrian army's one, the Austrian soldiers, forced to
load while standing, became easy targets for the Prussians. In the battles
of June 26 through July 22, the Austrians lost 53,075 killed, wounded, or
missing to the Prussians' 16,632. By the end of the war, the breechloader
had firmly proven itself over the muzzle-loader. The Prussians also moved
to breech-loading horse and field artillery pieces made of steel in place of
the cast-bronze and wrought-iron ordnance used by other nations.
Grooving of barrels gave way to rifling, which imparted a spinning
motion to the projectile.[20]

Despite its technological advantage, the Dreyse rifle (15 mm, or .589
in) enjoyed only a brief period of ascendancy. At Gravelotte, where
188,000 Germans fought 112,000 Frenchmen on August 18, 1870, the
pride of Germany's officer corps was swept away by the lighter, long-range
chassepot rifle (11 mm, or .432 in). While the Prussian needle-fire rifle

proved effective at six hundred yards, the chassepot killed at sixteen hundred yards. More than twenty thousand German officers and men died in this single battle. Two decades later, during civil war in Chile in 1891, the Männlicher rifle fired an eight-millimeter projectile of higher velocity and power of perforation than any other weapon of the day. Unlike older rifles, which when fired at great distances had little destructive effect, the Mannlicher could punch a hole through almost any vessel, bone, or tissue in its path. As a result, the new weapon reversed the casualty ratio for long-distance projectiles.[21]

In the period from the late eighteenth century to the Great War, military weaponry had evolved through various technologies, including the rifled bore, which put spin to the bullet; the gradual evolution from a rounded bullet to the elongated shape; and the change in the round nose to the sharply pointed spitzer nose. The trend toward the infliction of injury at greater distances through increased missile velocity forced a rethinking of the missile-casualty cases and a new look at the apparent anomalies seen by medical personnel unacquainted with the mechanics of wound formation. Frequently, for example, military surgeons saw small entrance and exit holes in the skin of a gunshot casualty and concluded that the internal damage was correspondingly slight. Given the realities of the high-velocity bullet and the effect known as *yaw*, the damage was in reality far more extensive than initially assumed. The spin imparted to the bullet by rifling had a negligible effect in stabilizing the missile when the increased mass in the tail of the bullet operated to increase the yaw. Moreover, in rapid-fire weapons, bullets were less subject to stabilization because of the heat-induced expansion of the barrel. This, too, contributed to excessive yaw in the missile.[22]

The yaw, which represented a deviation of the longitudinal axis from the line of flight, increased the amount of kinetic energy entering into the wound. Yaw did not occur with the muskets and smoothbore guns of the seventeenth and eighteenth centuries since, to have a yaw, the bullet had to have a length greater than its diameter. With the change in bullet dimensions and with the increase in velocity came an explosive effect in tissue destruction, even from the penetration of small fragments. And on entering different mediums (moving from air to tissue, from tissue to bone, and again from bone to tissue) the gyrations of a bullet and all of its motions became more exaggerated. The kinetic energy lost by a high-velocity bullet through retardation resulted in enormous destruction, tissue pulping, and bone shattering as the wound absorbed the impact.[23]

By 1885, most firearms had become lighter yet more deadly as armies moved to smokeless powder and to magazine or rapid-fire guns in place of single-loaders. At the same time, bullets of smaller caliber and with a harder metal jacket replaced the soft lead bullets of earlier weapons. This change resulted in projectiles that produced smaller wounds. Also, military physicians assumed that firing destroyed any pathogenic organisms on the bullet. This belief in a comparatively "clean" wound prevailed throughout the Boer War and carried into the trenches of France and Belgium in the early months of the Great War.[24]

From firelocks and wheel locks, to flintlocks, percussion locks, muzzle-loaders, and breechloaders, the range and rapidity of firepower increased remarkably in the nineteenth century. When combined with other improvements, such as rifling, brass-covered cartridges, smokeless powder, magazine feeding of cartridges, and machine guns, armies had available a combination of greater accuracy and dependability of weaponry, increased range and speed of fire, and improved concealment. Battles could now begin at longer ranges, and revised tactics forced companies of men to advance by short rushes, as well as in support groups spread out in artillery formation, with wider frontages and increased opportunity to turn the enemy's flank.[25] Paul F. Straub's *Medical Service in Campaign* (1910) gave clear recognition to the influence that the range and efficiency of the newer firearms had upon the medical service in battle. Not only was the character of the wounds largely determined by the trajectory, range, and penetration of the modern rifle bullet, but the disposition and uses of the medical department units were as well. Straub recognized that, while the wounds inflicted by modern weaponry were less severe than those from the old large-caliber muskets, their greater range and efficiency made rescue and removal of the wounded more difficult. Little difference existed among the military rifles adopted by countries in terms of their caliber, velocity, or range (see table 4.1).[26]

Table 4.1

COUNTRY	CALIBER	SIGHTING RANGE
United States	.300	2,850 yards
Great Britain	.303	2,786 yards
Austria	.315	2,187 yards
France	.315	2,187 yards
Germany	.311	2,187 yards
Japan	.256	2,187 yards
Spain	.275	2,187 yards
Russia	.300	2,096 yards

Changes in firearms—especially in the caliber and velocity of small weaponry—intensified the armament competition in the last decades of the nineteenth and early years of the twentieth centuries. By 1914, rifles had an approximate maximum range of five thousand yards. The point-blank danger range for a bullet fired at a soldier, where the trajectory was not higher than sixty-eight inches, was six hundred yards, that is, with the rifle firing directly at a target. More distant targets required elevating the rifle above the height of the average soldier. During a firefight on level terrain, the danger zone extended to nearly two thousand yards (see table 4.2).[27]

Table 4.2

	SIGHTING HEIGHT	POINT-BLANK DANGER SPACE
Firing position	Inches from Ground	Yards
Standing	56	718.6
Kneeling	30	629.4
Lying Down	12	589.7

Increased firepower changed the distribution of casualties by encompassing larger areas to the rear of the battle line. Infantry casualties, which before had extended 200 yards during volley-firing close-platoon formations, had now extended to 900 yards, with most occurring between 500 and 600 yards. At the closer ranges, the explosiveness of high-velocity projectiles meant severe wounds and massive hemorrhaging; at ranges greater than four hundred yards, except for penetrations of the larger bones or vital organs, wounds were serious but medically manageable.[28]

Hoping to mitigate the severities of warfare, delegates from seventeen European nations denounced the use of explosive bullets under the weight of four hundred grams in the Declaration of Saint Petersburg in 1868. At The Hague in 1899, however, Great Britain refused to concur in an agreement requiring all bullets to be encased in hard jackets. Basing their rationale on the Chitral campaign of 1895 and the need for a more effective stopping power, both England and the United States refused to sign the declaration. By the time of The Hague Peace Conference of 1907, only the United States had not assented to the agreement. Ironically, the diplomats who struggled to place restrictions on explosive and expanding bullets ignored the severity of wounds caused by high-explosive shells, machine guns, and high-velocity bullets, which were pointed instead of ogival and whose center of gravity was well back towards its base. The publication of Julius Fessler's research in 1905 on the effects of pointed bullets, as opposed to the more humane wound caused by the blunt-nosed, small-bore, cylindrical bullet, seemed to go unnoticed in diplomatic circles. One result of this ignorance was the tendency of the military to approach killing effectiveness on the basis of a "clean-killing" rather than the "clean-healing" ideal.[29]

Through the period of the American Civil War and the Franco-Prussian War, common practice placed medical assistance well beyond rifle range. This meant situating dressing stations five hundred or more yards to the rear of the line during the Civil War and up to three thousand yards behind the line in the Franco-Prussian War. With the introduction of small-caliber magazine rifles and long-range field pieces, sanitary planners realized that, if the wounded were to receive essential medical care, rescue and medical intervention would have to begin within the danger zone and during the course of battle.[30]

To the statisticians in the medical service, the range and effectiveness of modern rifles and artillery implied a level of casualties that required a significant rethinking of sanitary tactics and support. This became especially relevant given the increasing numbers of soldiers involved in battle (see table 4.3).[31]

Advances in military technology directly affected the evacuation of the sick and wounded, the level of available field surgery, and the types of wounds. Improvements in medical science, including advances in antiseptic surgery, meant that the ratio of killed to wounded diminished from previous wars', necessitating a larger medical staff. During the Franco-Prussian War, the German wounded numbered 116,821, or 14.8 percent of the total fighting force. Of this number, 17,300 died immediately, leaving nearly one hundred thousand requiring some level of medical treatment.

As a result of this experience, the German War Office anticipated a 20-percent casualty rate in future wars. For every seven thousand casualties, the War Office estimated twelve hundred killed; of the wounded, one-third would be seriously injured. The War Office anticipated larger numbers of men wounded by small arms, most of whom would be only temporarily disabled, provided they received early antiseptic treatment. This meant that, if treated close to the front lines, soldiers could return to the fighting line within fifteen to thirty days following an injury.[32] As a general practice, military planners seldom anticipated casualty rates exceeding 20 percent, excluding those killed outright. Of course, while the 20 percent covered the whole period of fighting, much higher percentages occurred at certain times or points in a given battle. For

Table 4.3

BATTLE	NATION	STRENGTH	PERCENTAGE KILLED/WOUNDED		RATIO KILLED/ WOUNDED
Shiloh	Union	62,682	2.670	13.40	1:4.8
1862	Confederate	40,335	4.270	19.80	1:4.6
Antietam	Union	56,000	3.749	16.93	1:4.5
1862	Confederate	40,000	6.700	21.93	1:3.2
Chickamauga	Union	58,222	2.800	16.70	1:5.9
1863	Confederate	66,366	3.400	22.00	1:6.4
Wilderness	Union	101,895	2.200	11.80	1:5.3
1864	Confederate	61,025	—	—	—
Spicheren	German	28,000	2.900	12.70+	1:4.3
1870	French	20,000	1.600	8.00+	1:5.2
Mars-la-Tour	German	66,300	2.900	12.70+	1:3.1
1870	French	126,170	1.080	8.00+	1:7.4
Gravelotte	German	146,000	3.040	10.37	1:3.8
1870	French	125,000	0.900	5.37	1:5.8
Sedan	German	165,400	0.989	3.91	1:3.9
1870	French	108,000	2.760	12.97	1:4.6
Yalu	Russian	21,000	3.000	5.60	1:2.0
1904	Japanese	40,966	0.500	2.00	1:4.0
Liao-yang	Russian	140,000	1.799	9.85	1:5.5
1904	Japanese	125,000	3.837	14.00+	1:4.0
Mukden	Russian	310,000	2.900	16.30+	1:5.4
1905	Japanese	340,000	4.410	17.64	1:4.0

example, during a twenty-minute period at Gravelotte, a German Fusilier Battalion experienced a 53-percent casualty rate; and, at Magersfontein, the Black Watch suffered 35-percent casualties, although the total loss of troops engaged in the battle numbered only 7.4 percent.[33]

Strategists predicted severe, often fatal wounds in the head, thigh, or shoulder areas and comparatively minor medical problems elsewhere. As C. H. Melville noted in 1894,

> Probably wounds of the large vessels of the limbs will tend to be more fatal, owing to the cleaner cutting action of the small-bore bullet; on the other hand, owing to the comparative absence of shock in a purely flesh wound by a small bullet, the wounded man should be more able to take measures to

control the hemorrhage of any vessel distally to the upper third of the thigh or upper arm. I would venture to predict then that, at the range where the decisive fire-fight is carried on, wounds will tend to be fatal, or moderately severe only; and that very severe or severe wounds will not commonly come under treatment. At the longer ranges wounds will more and more tend to be slight, owing to the diminishing momentum of the light bullet, and the comparatively high penetrating power conferred by its diminished calibre.[34]

Those involved in the planning of sanitary support referred frequently to the Manchurian campaign to illustrate the degree to which additional transport was needed to support the sick and wounded. Using this campaign as their benchmark, statisticians devised formulas to estimate the kind and amount of transportation required after battle. Military planners accompanied this casualty information with statistics regarding the time and material required for removal of sick and wounded men. For example,

$$M = \frac{W \times t}{T \times n}$$

determined the transport required in a given time to evacuate wounded to any point. Here, M represented the units of transport matériel (ambulances, carts, wagons, etc.) required or available; W, the number of sick and wounded; t, the time taken by the transport matériel to make one journey and return; T, the time allowed; and n, the number of patients each unit carried. With this formula, planners could anticipate the number of wagons required for recumbent or seated wounded. Planners developed similar calculations for other needs as well.[35]

Writing for *Military Surgeon* in 1912, Major J. H. Ford predicted that large units in a firefight would lose, on average, 12 percent each day. This meant twenty-four hundred casualties in a division, of whom perhaps 28 percent would be killed outright or would be too seriously injured to move. The remaining 1,728 required some level of accommodation. If an estimated sixty sick were added to this number, a total of 8.9 percent of the unit would require medical evacuation each battle day. These projected statistics also necessitated efficient evacuation of field hospitals to accommodate ongoing division losses over several days of fighting. Confusion or inability to accommodate wounded, Ford predicted, would result in serious morale problems for the army.[36]

As the size of armies increased, strategists predicted a million or more combatants on the field of battle. Well before the Great War, planners anticipated battlefield casualties in excess of one hundred forty thousand.

These predictions of massive battlefield fronts and accompanying casualties challenged the very basis of existing medical evacuation systems. At the heart of this challenge was the question of whether wounded men should lie unattended on the battlefield because of increased vulnerability to medical units or whether such units should attempt immediate relief regardless of the human cost.[37]

REASSESSMENT

As a result of the provisions in the Geneva Convention and the influence of the International Red Cross Society, litter bearers wearing the Red Cross badge on their left arm could claim immunity from capture. This, however, was their only privilege. Bearers still faced risks in the field as they exposed themselves to even greater dangers than faced by the fighting soldier. Given the destructive power of the newer weaponry, Austrian Surgeon Theodor Billroth (1829–94) questioned the effectiveness of existing medical evacuation systems. "We must come to the conclusion," he remarked, "that in future it will be no longer possible to remove the wounded from the field during the battle by means of bearers, since every man of them would be shot down, as bearers would be more exposed than men in the fighting-line; and the most that can be aimed at is that the wounded man of the future shall be attended to within twenty-four hours."[38] The surgeon general of the Prussian army, Adolf Bardeleben (1819–95), made a similar observation.

> Some urge an increase of bearers; but we must not forget that bearers have to go into the fire-line and expose themselves to the bullets. If we go on increasing their number, shall we not also be simply increasing the number of the wounded? The number of men provided for the transfer of the wounded now exceeds one thousand for each army corps. It is no true humanity that, in order to effect an uncertain amount of saving human life, a number of lives of other men should be sacrificed. The whole system of carrying away the wounded on litters during the battle must be abandoned, for it is altogether impracticable.[39]

Thus, with the increased range of modern weaponry, ambulance support came under serious examination. In earlier wars, ambulance bearers could move the wounded soldier to a collection station within five hundred yards of the place where he had fallen. With the increased range and effectiveness of the modern rifle, the distance of the collection station increased to twelve hundred yards. War correspondent Archibald Forbes, observing the loss of bearers and surgeons in the Franco-Prussian and Russo-Turkish wars, believed along with Billroth and Bardeleben that medical evacuation procedures required total renovation. "In the warfare of the future," Forbes predicted, "the service as now existing will be found utterly impracticable, since, with the improved man-killing appliances certain to be brought into action, the first battle would bodily wipe out the bearer organization carried on under fire."[40]

The Russo-Japanese war of 1904–5 illustrated the concern for stretcher-bearers in modern warfare. The collection of wounded from the battlefield proved to be especially dangerous in this war, with stretcher-bearers drawing heavy fire when attempting to move felled soldiers from the fighting line during the day. Moreover, sanitary personnel found it difficult to establish dressing stations in open country since they often drew enemy artillery fire; the enemy too often mistook the movement of stretcher-bearers and wounded for troop movement. In fighting over open terrain, the distance between the firing point and the point of impact became all too expansive with modern weaponry. The idea of protecting medical units under the neutrality of the Red Cross flag was all but lost. As one officer noted, "the Geneva Convention did not seem to have much application except in the case of captured Hospitals and Establishments such as those at Mukden. Indeed, it is doubtful if the Articles of the Convention go any further than this."[41]

Given these developments, strategists considered moving collecting stations further from the battle line to ensure relative safety for the wounded. This did not prove as simple as imagined because the removal of stations one mile back from the fighting increased the distances traveled by stretcher detachments and increased as well their exposure to hostile fire. And when sanitary personnel pushed the dressing station back nearly three miles from the fighting line, the extra distance required of the wagons and teams only multiplied their exhaustion and suscep-tibility to injury. The question was whether any real advantages were gained from rapid removal of the wounded or whether it only increased the number of casualties.[42]

Not all strategists believed that, under these new conditions, the collecting station remained a relevant part of the field ambulance system. Major T. P. Jones, writing in the *Journal of the Royal Army Medical Corps* in 1904, noted that the collecting station "must be regarded as obsolete." The battle-fields of modern warfare, he argued, spread over such a wide front that collecting the wounded in any one place prior to transportation to the dress-ing station no longer seemed practicable. It simply added to the suffering of the wounded and increased the work of the bearers. Instead, Jones urged the military to place dressing stations as close to the front as feasible. Although unintended, these strategic planners anticipated the impact of trench warfare in the placement of both collecting and dressing stations.[43]

In reviewing their options, medical planners also considered the effect wounded soldiers produced on the morale of comrades if not removed quickly from the field. In response to this dilemma, physicians and surgeons chose to administer morphine liberally to quiet the wounded. Equally important, planners addressed the need for instructing each soldier in first aid, particularly in checking hemorrhage and understanding the rationale for remaining in a sheltered area near the enemy rather than moving immediately to the rear.[44]

At the turn of the century, sanitary personnel in the American army accounted for 4.9 percent of the mobile-force strength. Of this number, 34.7 percent remained on active duty with the troops, while the balance served with the sanitary units themselves. Of those serving in the sanitary units, 37.2 percent were in the ambulance companies, 21.3 percent in the field hospitals. In the French army, the statistics were similar: sanitary personnel numbered 5.6 percent of the mobile forces, of which 37.2 percent were on duty with the regiments and the balance with the sanitary units. The German army devoted 6.58 percent of its personnel to the sanitary service, of which 30 percent remained on duty with the troops. The balance divided between the ambulance or bearer companies and the field hospitals.[45]

The military did not always approve of this division of responsibility. Some objected to removing men from combat ranks to serve as bearers. They disapproved of what they perceived as a divided command, noting that officers did not like to part with company bearers during battle. Moreover, they opposed mixing combatants and noncombatants in medical relief. Those who favored removing the bearer companies reasoned that this merely increased the numbers within the hospital corps who remained idle between battles.[46]

To supplement medical support, Red Cross societies organized auxiliaries to assist in evacuating the wounded. Though under military control during the war, they seldom worked closer to the battlefield than the field hospital. Usually they worked at stationary medical units at the base and on the lines of communication, thereby freeing regular military personnel for service closer to the battlefield. At the Geneva Convention in 1884, however, Sir Thomas Longmore insisted that, while armies appreciated medical volunteers, they had to be incorporated within the military establishment and subject to military regulations and command. Any other arrangement impeded an organized military operation.[47]

AMBULANCE DOGS

One innovation resulting directly from the increased range of modern weaponry was the use of dogs to search for wounded men. The idea originated with the monks of the Saint Bernard Hospice, who trained the well-known Saint Bernard dog to rescue travelers lost in the snow. Drawing upon this tradition, the German military trained dogs for messenger and outpost duty and trained them to search for the wounded. Although a fitful effort to use dogs was initiated in the Franco-Prussian War, the German army began in earnest in 1885. By 1890, trained sanitary-service dogs assigned to the Battalion of the Garde Jaeger were equipped with waterproof canvas packs, holding bandages, biscuits, a small cask of brandy or rum, and a bell. If the soldier was too weak to use the provisions, the dogs were trained to bark loudly for the stretcher-bearers.

With the aid of the German government, a society called the *Deutsche Verein für Sanitätshunde* (Society for the Training of Sanitary Dogs) organized at Oberdollendorf in 1893. In 1904, the Russians reported success with several dogs that the society had loaned to the Russian army. An exhibition held by the society in 1895 demonstrated the effective use of dogs in searching for the wounded. In England, a Major Richardson of the British Forty-fifth Regiment popularized the use of dogs, using a breed of collie crossed with retriever and setter. However, many different breeds proved effective in finding wounded men. Russia chose the dog of the Caucasus, Austria the Dalmatian, Turkey the Asiatic sheepdog, Germany the collie and Airedale, and France used crossbreeds.[48]

By 1912, ambulance dogs were common to almost all of Europe's armies. Typically, the military attached two dogs to each ambulance company. In tests in Germany and England, dogs proved especially effective in discovering soldiers overlooked on the battlefield. Dogs were used by Germany in the Boxer rebellion, by the British in South Africa, by the French in Algiers, and by the Russians during actions in Manchuria. Similar uses were made by Austria, Italy, Switzerland, Holland, and the United States.

At the outbreak of the Great War, Germany had more than two thousand dogs in its sanitary corps. Trained by the German Red Cross, these dogs were used successfully in the Vosges, the Argonne Forest, and other heavily wooded regions. The military eventually employed dogs in trench warfare; adapting to the nature of a stationary war, dogs even carried ropes to the wounded in front of the trenches, enabling the wounded soldier to be pulled to safety without endangering the lives of sanitary corpsmen.[49]

"Self-propelled" Ambulances

The development of the automobile (and later the airplane) profoundly changed the art of war and, with it, the collection and evacuation of wounded. Nations tested motorized transportation in almost every branch of military service. Recognizing its potential significance, the German emperor offered a twenty-thousand-dollar prize in 1901 for the best motorized design for general military use; a year later, the British War Office made a similar offer.[50]

The British tested steam-propelled automobiles in the South African veldts and in 1901 directed that the Mechanical Transport Committee test various types of lorries. The French army demonstrated a motorized staff vehicle during maneuvers in 1898 and a steam-propelled surgeon's wagon as a field hospital. The Straker-Squire ambulance van (1906–8) became the first motorized ambulance used by the British army. Tested in summer maneuvers in 1907, it was attached to the military hospital at Oxford and operated between there and military corps at Thames and Aylesbury. By 1912–13, the *Service de Santé* (French Army Medical Service) had introduced the Boulant vehicle (1912–18) with a fully equipped mobile surgery unit using the same chassis as the Paris bus. Containing a full operating theater twelve feet by seven feet, complete with table and electric light, the Boulant had the appearance of the earlier Moses ambulance, which when stationary had tenting that had unfolded from its sides to form additional shelter for patients awaiting attention or recuperating from surgery.[51]

American development of self-propelled vehicles lagged behind that of Europe. Nevertheless, the War Department *Annual Reports* for 1895 did argue for the equipping of a regiment with motorized vehicles in order to test their utility.[52] In 1900, the United States Signal Corps experimented with electric-powered vehicles and found them unsatisfactory because of their weight, their limited range, and the difficulty of recharging their batteries. A similar test of both steam and internal-combustion engines occurred in 1901, with the Signal Corps concluding that the internal-combustion engine was preferable to either the steam or the electric vehicle because it required less fuel and water.[53]

Notwithstanding this recommendation, medical planners initially considered steam-propelled vehicles more practical because of their lack of vibration, the availability of fuel and water, and their need for fewer parts and repairs.[54] In general, the military concluded that the motorized ambulance was less expensive than animal-driven vehicles. Over time, an economy of resources accrued; although initial start-up costs remained high, the continued upkeep of wagons and horses made investment in the motorized ambulance more cost-effective. In contrast, the cost of transporting horses and mules long distances—and their susceptibility to disease and climate—diminished their effectiveness.[55]

Although roads near the front were often little more than "mire and rut," with appropriate rope and tackle support the motorized ambulance could travel through muddy areas more dependably than could conventional wagons drawn by horses or mules. The Hawey car used by the Royal Army Medical Corps carried twelve patients between the evacuation hospital and the advanced base at a speed of thirty miles an hour. With its speed and dependability, the motorcar greatly improved the ability of the R.A.M.C. to maintain steady evacuation toward base hospitals and to replenish medical supplies in field hospitals.[56]

Tests performed by the Quartermaster's Department of the U.S. Army in 1906 at the Washington Barracks with a Ruger ambulance body mounted on a White steam-motor chassis resulted in the later purchase of six cars powered by internal-combustion engines. By 1912, the American army had authorized motor ambulances for use at Letterman General Hospital, Fort Riley, Fort Leavenworth, Fort D. A. Russell, and Fort Bayard. Because of repeated breakdowns, however, medical officers were initially reluctant to urge the adoption of motorized ambulances within the ambulance service. This attitude eventually changed as a result of improvements in designs and construction, the development of more dependable machines, the extensive motorization of European armies, road improvements, and more successful field tests. By 1913, the United States Army stood prepared to make a major investment in motorized transport.

During the U.S.–Mexican border activities, the United States mobilized a division of regulars at San Antonio in 1911, supporting it with a sanitary train of four field hospitals and ambulance companies. With the subsequent occupation of Vera Cruz in 1913, the brigade in Texas City was accompanied by a field hospital but no ambulance company. This circumstance changed in 1917 when twelve thousand soldiers moved into Mexico under Brigadier General John "Black Jack" Pershing, accompanied by two motorized ambulance companies and two field hospitals. The campaign gave the Medical Department valuable experience in sanitary formations that had previously existed only in theory. More importantly, the expedition tested the capability of the motorized ambulance company and provided important information on sanitary tactics for America's eventual entry into the First World War.[57]

In August 1914, the Medical Department sent a motor ambulance to an ambulance company at Texas City; by October of the same year, motor ambulances were in use at fourteen posts and hospitals. In July 1915, a board of medical officers recommended to the surgeon general the extensive use of motorized vehicles in the ambulance service. But not until

1916 during the army's punitive expedition into Mexico did the War Department recognize the full significance of motorized transport. This experience led to a recommendation that three-fourths of the transportation required to support medical units be by motor vehicles. By July 1917, the Quartermaster's Department had acquired 2,965 motortrucks, 58 motor tank trucks, 12 motor machine-shop trucks, 6 motor wrecking trucks, 430 automobiles, and 670 motorcycles.[58]

Impediments aside, most countries recognized the significance of the motorized ambulance in terms of service, speed of evacuation, and dependability. Several nations, including France, Austria, Germany, Russia, and Switzerland, subsidized automobile organizations, paying car owners a stipend each year on the condition that, in the event of war, their vehicles would be available for military use. The intent was clearly to offset the cost of purchasing fleets of vehicles during peacetime. The military subsidized car owners for a period of five years, or the average life of the vehicle. Membership in these subsidized automobile organizations was voluntary except in Austria. The military also recognized the importance of electric streetcars, traction engines (Renard-type), industrial vehicles, tourist cars, limousines, and buses as valuable conveyances during war.[59]

Although the military subsidy program worked well for Europe's armies, neither it nor the concept of the Volunteer Motor Corps fit with American policies or traditions. Instead, the War Department concluded that motorized ambulance vehicles should be assimilated into the National Guard or the Federal Reserve.[60]

On the eve of the Great War, Europe stood poised to support its armies with a combination of animal and machine power. From more traditional mule power to dhoolies, camel support, oxcarts, hand transports, and motor ambulances, medical evacuation systems reflected the experiences of Europe's countless wars. Military planners hoped that such innovations as ambulance dogs, electric lights, bicycles, and motorized vehicles would bridge the expanded battlefield anticipated in future wars. Except for the English—who seemed at times more content to view the future from the perspective of an aging empire—Europe's armies stood open to experimentation. Few, however, foresaw the magnitude of the impending war and the demands that soon would be required of medical evacuation systems. Here again, experience would serve as the lightning rod to change.

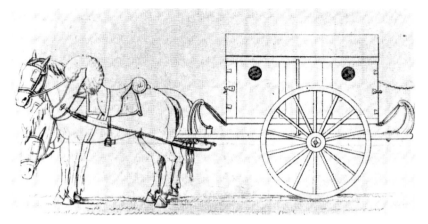

1. Larrey's two-wheeled ambulance. Dominique-Jean Larrey, *Mémoires de chirurgie/militarie, et campagnes* (4 vols.; Paris: J. Smith, 1812–17), I, plate 3.

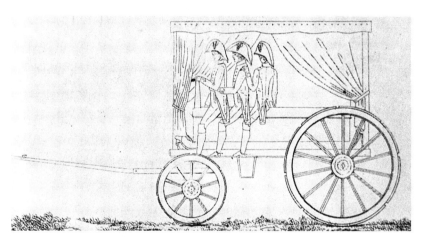

2. Percy's surgical wagon. Dominique-Jean Larrey, *Mémoires de chirurgie militaire, et campagnes* (4 vols.; Paris: J. Smith, 1812–17), I, plate 6.

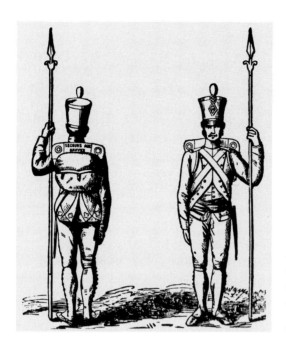

3. Percy's stretcher-bearers in marching order.
George J. H. Evatt, *Ambulance Organization, Equipment, and Transport* (London: William Clowes, 1886), 43.

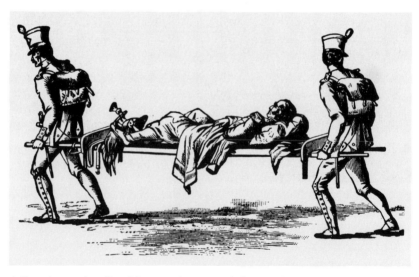

4. Percy's stretcher fitted for carrying wounded men. George J. H. Evatt, *Ambulance Organization, Equipment, and Transport* (London: William Clowes, 1886), 43.

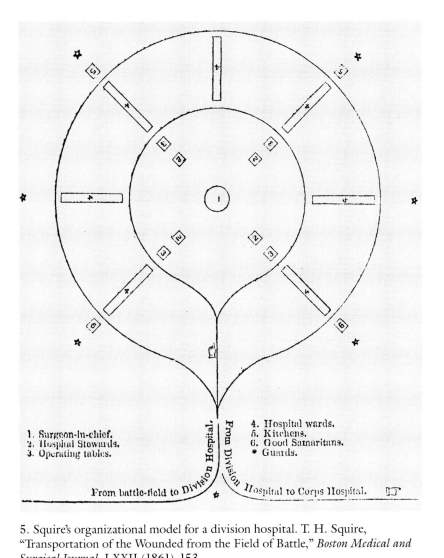

1. Surgeon-in-chief.
2. Hospital Stewards.
3. Operating tables.

4. Hospital wards.
5. Kitchens.
6. Good Samaritans.
* Guards.

From battle-field to Division Hospital.

From Division Hospital to Corps Hospital.

5. Squire's organizational model for a division hospital. T. H. Squire, "Transportation of the Wounded from the Field of Battle," *Boston Medical and Surgical Journal*, LXXII (1861), 153.

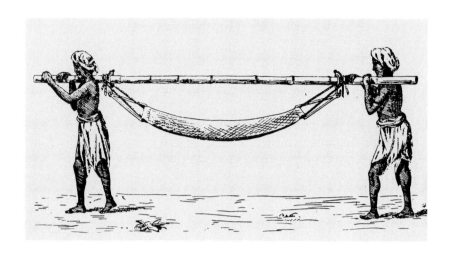

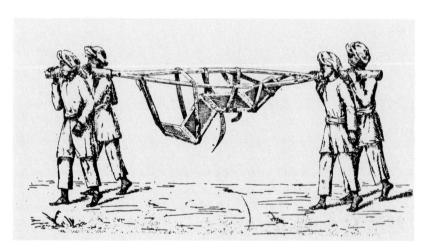

6. The common dandy (*top*) and Bareilly dandy (*bottom*). [Anonymous], "Dandies for Field Service," *Indian Medical Gazette*, V (1870), 257.

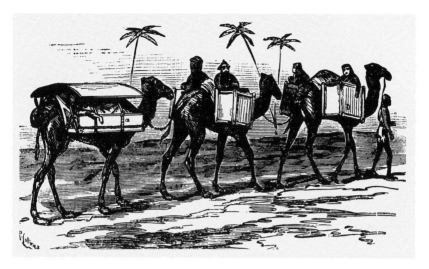

7. A convoy of sick in camel kujjawas and a camel dhoolie. George J. H. Evatt, *Ambulance Organization, Equipment, and Transport* (London: William Clowes, 1886), 60.

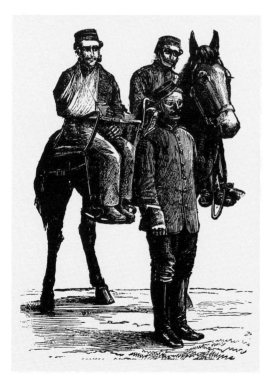

8. Mule cacolets or chairs. George J. H. Evatt, *Ambulance Organization, Equipment, and Transport* (London: William Clowes, 1886), 57.

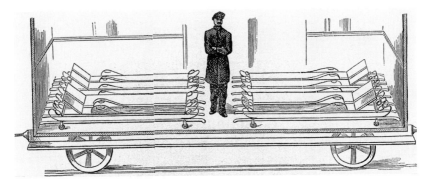

9. A freight car fitted with eight spring-bed stretchers. George A. Otis, *A Report on a Plan for Transporting Wounded Soldiers by Railway in Time of War, with Descriptions of Various Methods Employed for This Purpose on Different Occasions* (Washington, D.C.: Surgeon General's Office, 1875), 28.

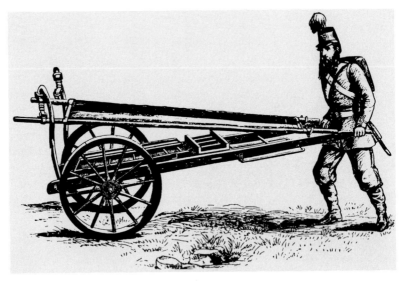

10. The China wheelbarrow ambulance. Thomas Longmore, "Report on the Fitness for Use in the British Service of a Wheeled Ambulance Transport Conveyance," *Army Medical Department Report*, London, VII (1865), opposite 506.

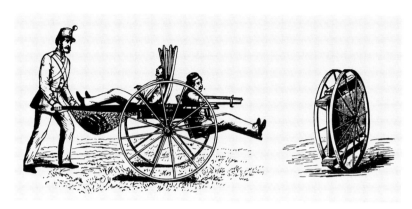

11. Neudörfer's two-wheeled litter, open for wounded transport, packed for carriage. Thomas Longmore, "Report on the Fitness for Use in the British Service of a Wheeled Ambulance Transport Conveyance," *Army Medical Department Report*, London, VII (1865), opposite 509.

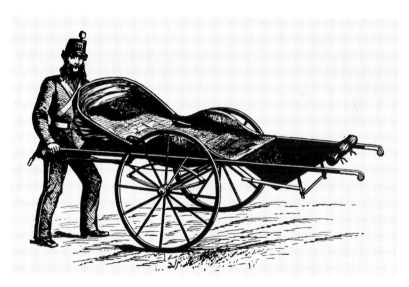

12. Neuss's two-wheeled litter. Thomas Longmore, "Report on the Fitness for Use in the British Service of a Wheeled Ambulance Transport Conveyance," *Army Medical Department Report*, London, VII (1865), opposite 508.

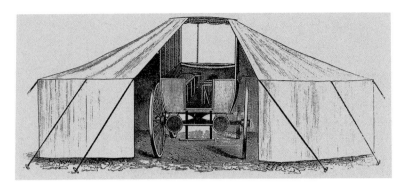

13. The Moses ambulance wagon and tent. United States Government, Surgeon General's Office, *The Medical and Surgical History of the War of the Rebellion*, part III, vol. II, *Surgical History* (Washington, D.C.: Government Printing Office, 1883), 945.

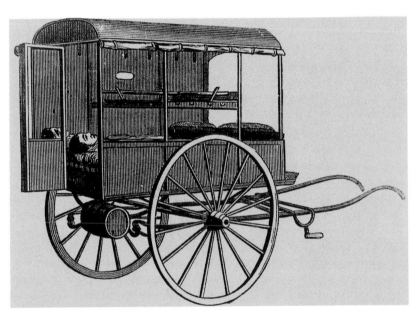

14. The Coolidge ambulance wagon. United States Government, Surgeon General's Office, *The Medical and Surgical History of the War of the Rebellion*, part III, vol. II, *Surgical History* (Washington, D.C.: Government Printing Office, 1883), 947.

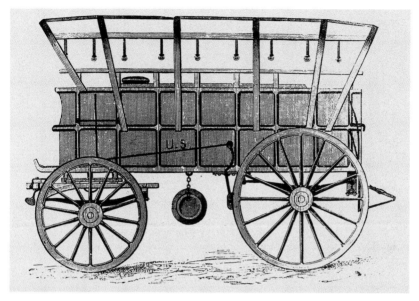

15. The Tripler ambulance wagon. United States Government, Surgeon General's Office, *The Medical and Surgical History of the War of the Rebellion*, part III, vol. II, *Surgical History* (Washington, D.C.: Government Printing Office, 1883), 947.

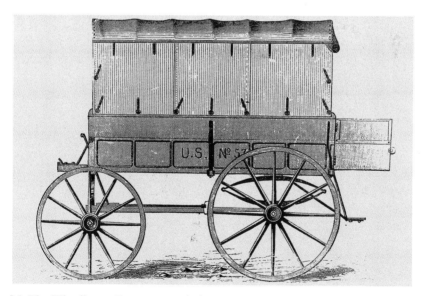

16. The Wheeling or Rosecrans ambulance wagon. United States Government, Surgeon General's Office, *The Medical and Surgical History of the War of the Rebellion*, part III, vol. II, *Surgical History* (Washington, D.C.: Government Printing Office, 1883), 948.

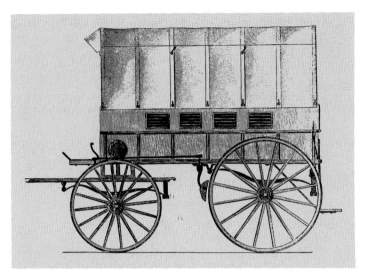

17. The Rucker ambulance wagon. United States Government, Surgeon General's Office, *The Medical and Surgical History of the War of the Rebellion*, part III, vol. II, *Surgical History* (Washington, D.C.: Government Printing Office, 1883), 952.

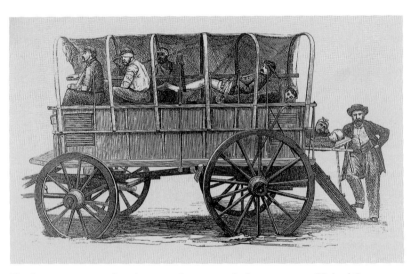

18. An army wagon fitted up as a Langer ambulance wagon. United States Government, Surgeon General's Office, *The Medical and Surgical History of the War of the Rebellion*, part III, vol. II, *Surgical History* (Washington, D.C.: Government Printing Office, 1883), 956.

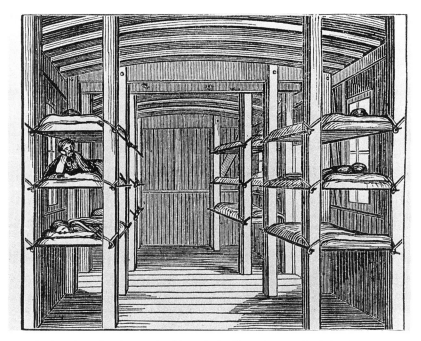

19. The interior of an improvised hospital railcar. George A. Otis, *A Report on a Plan for Transporting Wounded Soldiers by Railway in Time of War, with Descriptions of Various Methods Employed for This Purpose on Different Occasions* (Washington, D.C.: Surgeon General's Office, 1875), 6.

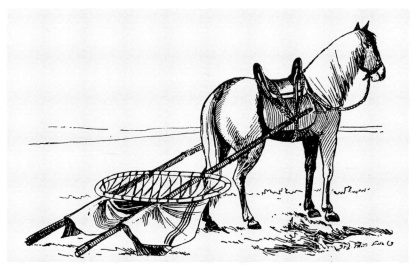

20. A Dakota Indian travois. John Van R. Hoff, "The Travois—A New Sanitary Appliance in the First Line of Battlefield Assistance," *Proceedings*, Association of Military Surgeons of the United States (1894), 73.

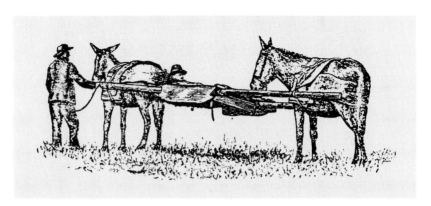

21. A wounded soldier conveyed on a double-mule litter. George A. Otis, *A Report to the Surgeon General on the Transport of Sick and Wounded by Pack Animals* (Washington, D.C.: Government Printing Office, 1877), 19.

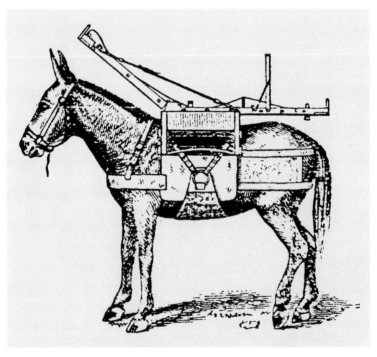

22. McElderry's single-mule litter. George A. Otis, *A Report to the Surgeon General on the Transport of Sick and Wounded by Pack Animals* (Washington, D.C.: Government Printing Office, 1877), 15.

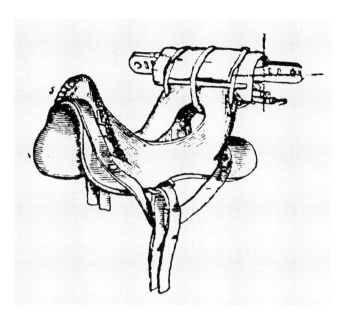

23. The Rooker saddle attachment packed to a McClellan saddle. George A. Otis, *A Report to the Surgeon General on the Transport of Sick and Wounded by Pack Animals* (Washington, D.C.: Government Printing Office, 1877), 13.

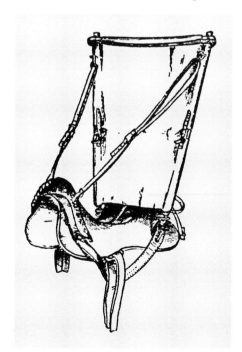

24. The Rooker saddle attachment for support of a wounded soldier. George A. Otis, *A Report to the Surgeon General on the Transport of Sick and Wounded by Pack Animals* (Washington, D.C.: Government Printing Office, 1877), 13.

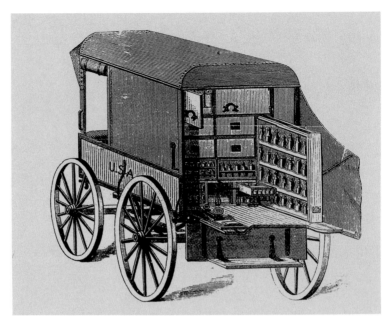

25. The Autenrieth medicine wagon. United States Government, Surgeon General's Office, *The Medical and Surgical History of the War of the Rebellion*, part III, vol. II, *Surgical History* (Washington, D.C.: Government Printing Office, 1883), 918.

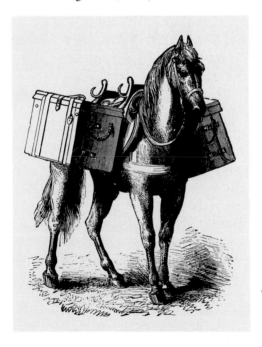

26. Medical supplies carried on a two-pack mule. George J. H. Evatt, *Ambulance Organization, Equipment, and Transport* (London: William Clowes, 1886), 54.

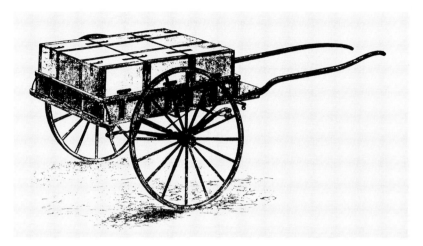

27. The U.S. Army medical transport cart. David L. Huntington and George A. Otis, "No. 6 Description of the U.S. Army Medical Transport Cart Model of 1876," *International Exhibition of 1876, Hospital of Medical Department, United States Army* (Philadelphia: n.p., 1876), 2.

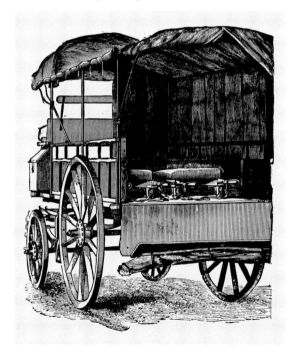

28. British army sick-transport wagon, showing the Faris stretcher on the floor of the wagon. George J. H. Evatt, *Ambulance Organization, Equipment, and Transport* (London: William Clowes, 1886), 72.

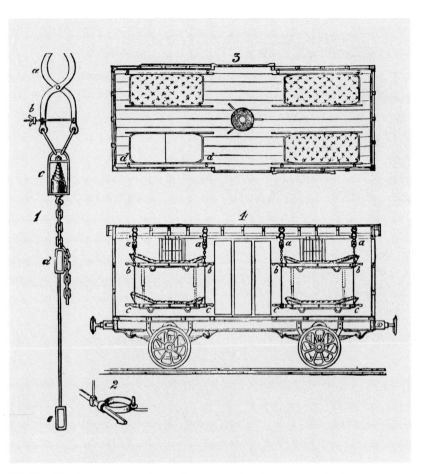

29. The Hamburg system of stretcher suspension in an improvised railcar. George J. H. Evatt, *Ambulance Organization, Equipment, and Transport* (London: William Clowes, 1886), 100.

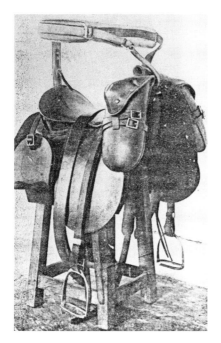

30. A saddle support for wounded cavalry. H. G. Hathaway, "Ambulance for Mounted Troops," *Proceedings*, Association of Military Surgeons of the United States, XIII (1903), 134.

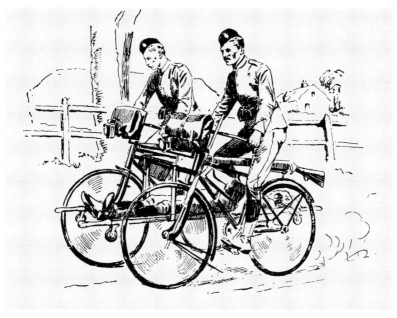

31. A bicycle ambulance. John S. Riddell, *A Manual of Ambulance* (London: Griffin, 1894), 164.

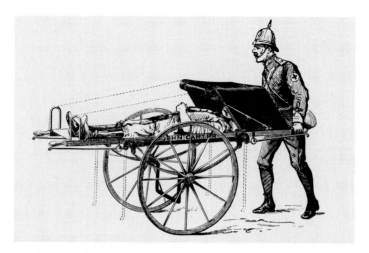

32. Carter's "simplex" ambulance. John S. Riddell, *A Manual of Ambulance* (London: Griffin, 1894), 162.

33. Apparatus for carrying a wounded man on a soldier's back. Thomas Longmore, "Report on Certain Conveyances for Use in Transporting Sick and Wounded from the Field of Action," *Army Medical Department Report*, London, VI (1866), 478.

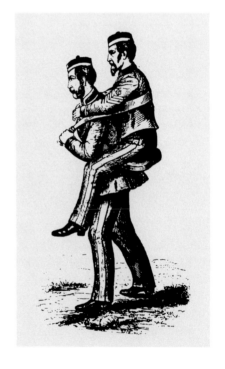

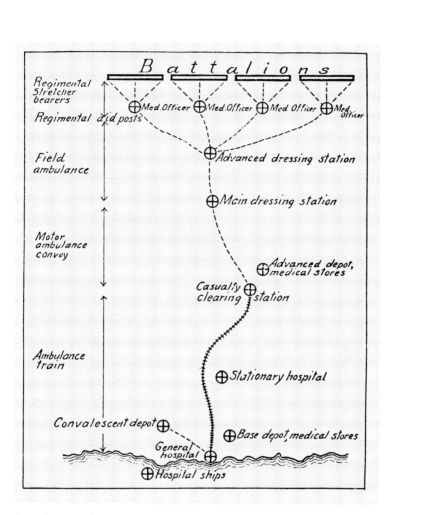

34. Diagram of the British army evacuation organization. W. W. Keen, *The Treatment of War Wounds* (Philadelphia: Saunders, 1917), 19.

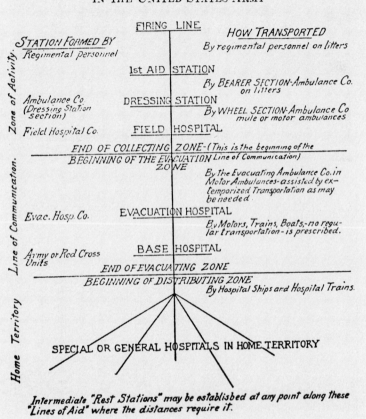

ZONES OF COLLECTION, EVACUATION, AND DISTRIBUTION IN THE UNITED STATES ARMY

FIRING LINE

HOW TRANSPORTED

STATION FORMED BY
Regimental personnel

By regimental personnel on litters

Zone of Activity.

1st AID STATION

By BEARER SECTION-Ambulance Co.
on litters

Ambulance Co.
(Dressing Station
section)

DRESSING STATION

By WHEEL SECTION-Ambulance Co.
mule or motor ambulances

Field Hospital Co.

FIELD HOSPITAL

END OF COLLECTING ZONE-(This is the beginning of the
BEGINNING OF THE EVACUATION Line of Communication)
ZONE

By the Evacuating Ambulance Co. in
Motor Ambulances-assisted by extemporized Transportation as may
be needed

Line of Communication.

Evac. Hosp. Co.

EVACUATION HOSPITAL

By Motors, Trains, Boats,-no regular transportation-is prescribed.

Army or Red Cross
Units

BASE HOSPITAL

END OF EVACUATING ZONE
BEGINNING OF DISTRIBUTING ZONE

By Hospital Ships and Hospital Trains.

Home Territory

SPECIAL OR GENERAL HOSPITALS IN HOME TERRITORY

Intermediate "Rest Stations" may be established at any point along these
"Lines of Aid" where the distances require it.

35. Diagram of the U.S. Army evacuation organization. W. W. Keen, *The Treatment of War Wounds* (Philadelphia: Saunders, 1917), 18.

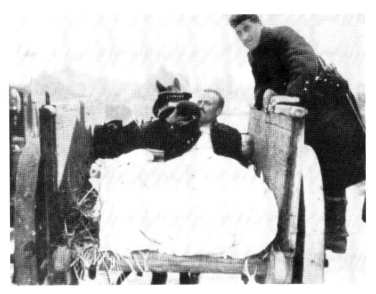

36. Two-wheeled farmcart. Archibald Magill Fauntleroy, *Report on the Medico-Military Aspects of the European War: From Observations Taken Behind the Allied Armies in France* (Washington, D.C.: Government Printing Office, 1915), opposite 43.

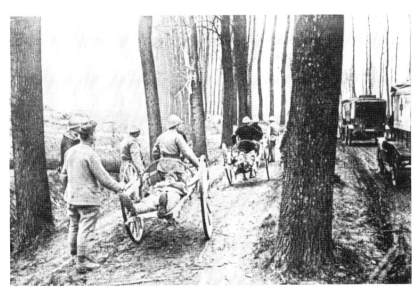

37. Stretchers slung between two wheels, leaving the trenches. American Ambulance Field Service, *Friends of France: The Field Service of the American Ambulance Described by Its Members* (Boston: Houghton Mifflin, 1916), opposite 156.

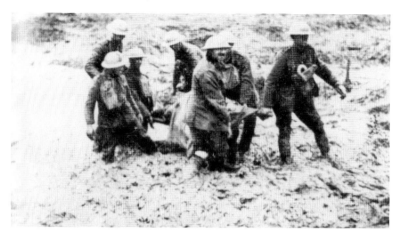

38. Stretcher-bearers returning from no-man's-land, Somme, 1916. Arthur
Graham Butler, *The Australian Army Medical Services in the War of 1914–
1918* (3 vols.; Canberra: Australian War Memorial, 1940), II, opposite 76.

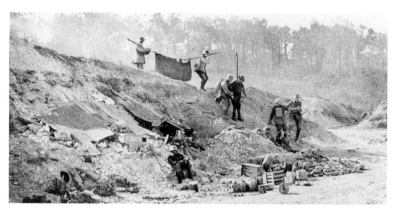

39. German prisoners carrying wounded men in a waterproof sheet, during fighting at Bray, August 22, 1918. Arthur Graham Butler, *The Australian Army Medical Services in the War of 1914–1918* (3 vols.; Canberra:
Australian War Memorial, 1940), II, opposite 295.

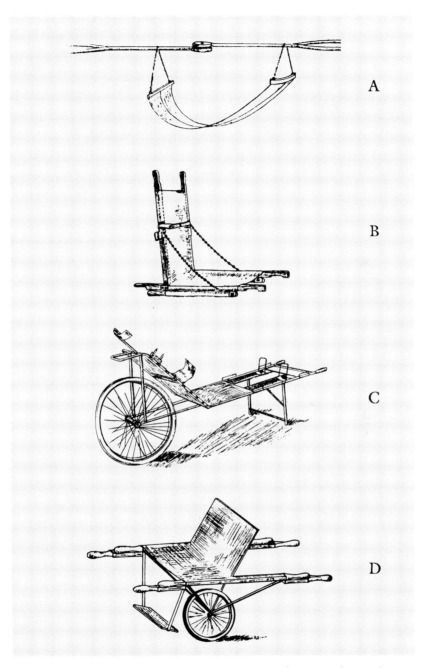

40. (a) Colt trench stretcher, (b) Willis stretcher, (c) Victor stretcher carrier, and (d) Blackham stretcher carrier. William G. Macpherson, *History of the Great War Based on Official Documents* (12 vols.; London: His Majesty's Stationery Office, 1924), IV, 581.

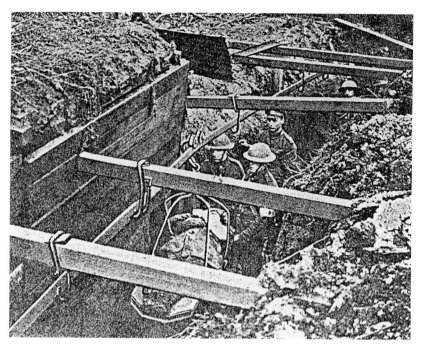

41. An overhead trench railway ambulance trolley. [Anonymous], "Transportation and Care of the Wounded at the Front," *Modern Hospital*, IX (1917), 444.

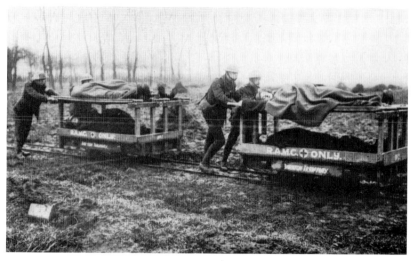

42. Ambulance cars on a temporary railway. John Gilmour, "Transportation of the Wounded," *Military Surgeon*, XLII (1918), opposite 8.

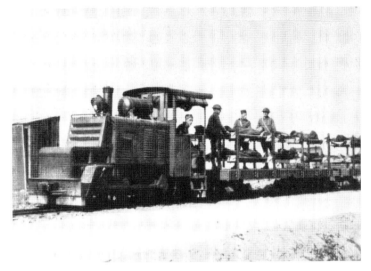

43. Decauville light-railway system fitted for carrying wounded soldiers. M. W. Ireland (ed.), *The Medical Department of the United States Army in the World War* (15 vols.; Washington, D.C.: Government Printing Office, 1925), VIII, 45.

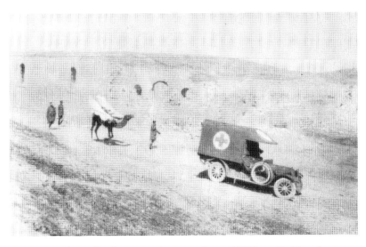

44. A camel cacolet for recumbent patients. William G. Macpherson, *History of the Great War Based on Official Documents* (12 vols.; London: His Majesty's Stationery Office, 1924), IV, 603.

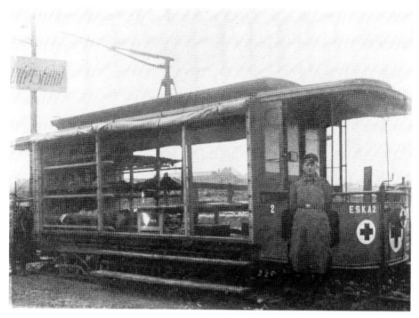

45. A German streetcar commandeered for transport of wounded, nine recumbent and sixteen sitting. General Surgeon Dr. Altgelt, "The Preparation for the Great German Offensive on the Western Front in the Spring of 1918, *Military Surgeon*, LIV (1924), opposite 605.

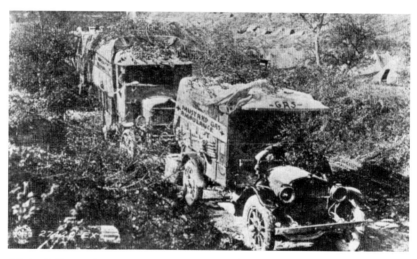

46. Ambulances for carrying mustard gas patients. These ambulances are parked until they can be demustardized. Note the camouflage used to render them less conspicuous to enemy aviators. H. L. Gilchrist, "Chemical Warfare and Its Medical Significance," *Military Surgeon*, LXIII (1928), 483.

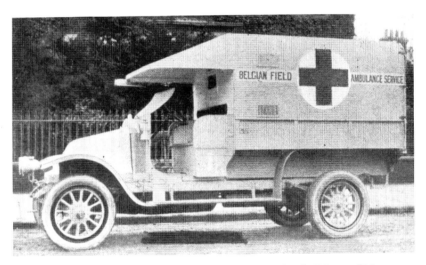

47. The Belgian field ambulance motorcar. F. L. Pleadwell, "Types of Motor Ambulances Observed Abroad," *Military Surgeon*, XLVII (1920), opposite 332.

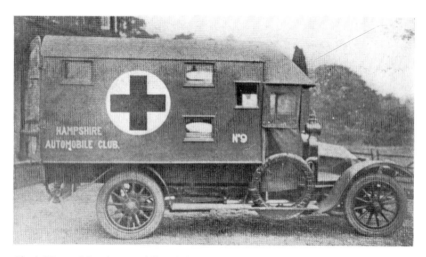

48. A Hampshire Automobile Club ambulance motorcar with three-ply wood sides, canvas top, and Hooper windows. Note protection given to the driver by the canvas cowl and side curtains. F. L. Pleadwell, "Types of Motor Ambulances Observed Abroad," *Military Surgeon*, XLVII (1920), opposite 332.

Owing to the fact that five new sections of ambulances have recently been sent to the front, the waiting list of the past eighteen months has been depleted, and accordingly a limited number of

Volunteer Ambulance Drivers are Wanted

New men are also needed from time to time to fill the places of those who return to America on leave, or who are unable to re-enlist at the expiration of their six months in the field.

REQUISITE QUALIFICATIONS

American Citizenship — Good Health — Clean Record — Ability to drive and repair Automobiles — Sufficient Funds to assume Travelling Expenses. (No salary, but living expenses paid.)

For further details and terms of service apply to

WILLIAM R. HEREFORD   or to   HENRY D. SLEEPER

Headquarters American Ambulance,   c/o Lee, Higginson & Co.,

14 Wall Street, New York   State Street, Boston

49. An advertisement for volunteer American ambulance drivers. American Ambulance Field Service, *Friends of France: The Field Service of the American Ambulance* (Boston: Houghton Mifflin, 1916), opposite index.

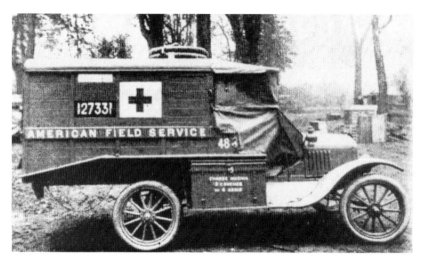

50. A Ford ambulance motorcar in the American Field Service. Note the top rack for spare tires and the side box for tools and extra gasoline. A. Piatt Andrew, "The Genesis of the American Ambulance Service with the French Army, 1915–1917," *Military Surgeon*, LVII (1925), opposite 363.

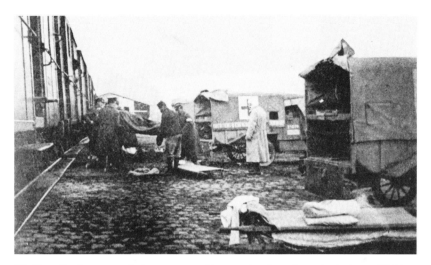

51. Transferring wounded men to a railway train. American Ambulance Field Service, *Friends of France: The Field Service of the American Ambulance* (Boston: Houghton Mifflin, 1916), opposite 158.

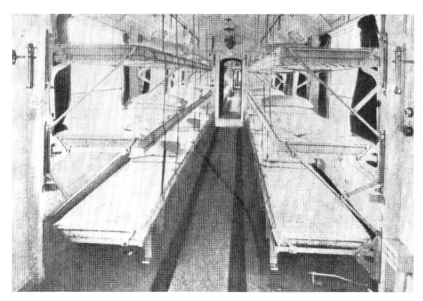

52. A ward railcar arranged for recumbent cases in a British ambulance train. F. L. Pleadwell, "British Ambulance Trains," *Military Surgeon*, XLVI (1920), opposite 56.

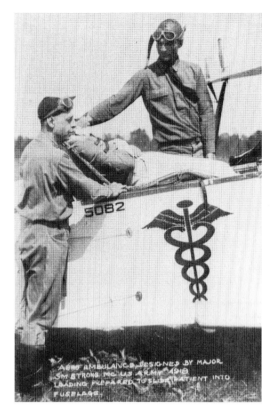

53. Loading a patient into the fuselage of an aeroambulance. S. M. Strong, "Aero Ambulance," *Military Surgeon*, XLIV (1919), opposite 363.

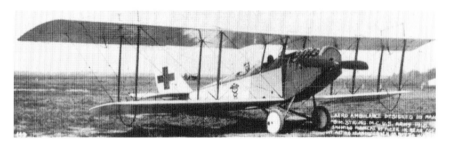

54. The aeroambulance designed by Major S. M. Strong. S. M. Strong, "Aero Ambulance," *Military Surgeon*, XLIV (1919), opposite 363.

PART THREE

The Great War

5

New Challenges

The Great War began as a war of movement, with German armies sweeping across Belgium in August 1914, sending shock waves through the capitals of Europe. By September, however, the German advance ground to an unexpected halt following the battle of the Marne (September 5–12). A race to the sea quickly followed, with the German and French armies attempting to outflank each other. At the end of the first battle of Ypres (October 30 to November 24), the western front entered into a stalemate, confined largely to trench warfare, which stretched from France to part of Belgium, from Switzerland to the North Sea. For a period of three years, this front, consisting of fifteen thousand miles of zigzag trenches several lines deep, seldom advanced in either direction more than ten miles at any point. As historian Russell F. Weigley explained, "The size of the armies soon determined that there would be no more flanks for would-be Napoléons to turn, and the war degenerated into a head-on exchange of assaults and casualties, with battle not an occasional climax but an almost continuous event, that has given the phrases 'the World War' and 'the Western Front' their ominous connotations."[1] Brigadier General William Mitchell in his *Memoirs of World War I: "From Start to Finish of Our Greatest War"* (1960), said it not too differently: "The art of war had departed. Attrition, or the gradual killing off of the enemy, was all the ground armies were capable of."[2]

NO-MAN'S-LAND

What had begun as a war of movement devolved gradually and demonstrably into a war of siege characterized by trench fighting; short, trench-by-trench attacks made under barrages; suicidal assaults against the entrenched power of machine guns; elaborate tunnel mining; brutal night skirmishes in no-man's-land; defensive barbed-wire entanglements; and moving walls of artillery fire that, during some battles, sent eighteen shells into each square yard of front. Opposing trenches ranged from several yards to five hundred or more yards apart, between which lay strips of barbed-wire entanglements and other obstructions. There, too, sprawled the bodies of those who had fallen in previous assaults, leaving "a veritable plague along certain parts of the line [which was] . . . largely responsible for the prevalence of flies close to the firing-line."[3] The reality of trench warfare added to the impersonalization of the violence. Between the opposing lines of men, concealed like rabbits, was a deserted land — a dead land — where fighting from a tactical point of view had little strategic outcome save the massing of guns, shells, and attackers against the superior effectiveness of defensive firepower.[4]

Differences in topography between the British and French zones make comparisons difficult. In general, however, the British trench system had three lines (front, support, and reserve), while the French had two lines (front and support). Each was built either above- or belowground in a zigzag pattern (about ten feet of straight trench, then an abrupt five-foot turn, followed by another ten feet of straight trench) to reduce the destructive effect of enfilade fire or shells falling into the trenches; the lines were joined by communication trenches, with entrance from an access trench in the rear. Unlike the French three-hundred-mile sector between the Somme and Switzerland (which was quiet through much of the war, especially the area between Nancy and the Swiss border), and unlike the Belgian fifteen-mile sector from Nieuport to the point north of the Ypres Salient, the British Commonwealth armies maintained an eighty-five-mile front from the Ypres Salient to the River Somme and chose to employ alternating pressure with continuous activity across the entire zone.

The Germans assumed a defensive posture after their failure to effect a breakthrough in October 1914; the stalemate became a reality in the spring of 1915. With their greater tactical use of machine guns and their commanding position on higher ground, the German army wreaked havoc against the offensive efforts of the French and British. German positions typically consisted of a wide area of low-lying ground that was trenched and wired, behind which massed troops in support trenches, with more in reserve. This defensive organization was supplemented by a line of machine guns positioned eight hundred yards apart in concrete strong points. Behind the front trenches rose ridge after ridge of higher ground that commanded miles of adjacent terrain. Examples included the Passchendaele, Messines, Aubers, and Vimy ridges. With their excellent system of ground observation, the Germans were able to inflict severe losses almost at will.[5]

New military technology had an immediate and devastating impact on the battlefields of the First World War. Of the 61 million troops from sixteen warring countries, 7.8 million were killed or died almost immediately of their wounds, 19.6 million were wounded, and another 7 million were missing or made prisoners of war. As one British observer keenly noted, "During the war, for the first time in the history of our army, commanders became millionaires in men and medical officers millionaires in casualties."[6]

The magnitude of this slaughter tested the organizational and conceptual strengths of each of the belligerent powers. The number of litters and litter bearers, the distance to be traveled by litter squads, and the time consumed for each loaded litter were factors critical to military strategy. So, too, were the problems of collecting casualties within each sector of the field, the distance to collecting and dressing stations, and the impediments of night work. Mobility remained the focus of an efficient ambulance-company service; and the variables of too much weight, proper shoeing of animals, forage, human and animal exhaustion, numbers of motor ambulances and traction motors, employment of civilian vehicles by rental or appropriation, and use of empty field wagons spelled the difference between a medical debacle and a successful evacuation. Statistical averages of the percentages killed (20 percent), those unable to bear transportation (8 percent), those able to be transported in a sitting position (20 percent), those requiring stretchers (12 percent), and those able to walk (40 percent) marked the parameters within which medical strategists did their planning.[7]

Medical evacuation directly affected the very basis of military tactics. During an advance, evacuation, as in defensive trench warfare, was a relatively simple task. In retreat, however, or in offensive operations across no-man's-land, conditions changed dramatically. Men unable to withstand being moved were sometimes left, along with attendants, to fall into the hands of the enemy. Even with the protection of the Geneva Convention, armies did not take lightly the decision to leave troops behind. Wounded soldiers on both sides feigned death or hid for fear of being "put to death by a merciful enemy." The gruesome fate that befell many of these men inevitably affected morale.[8]

Opposing armies were not immune to the Geneva Convention or to the collection of wounded under a white or Red Cross flag. The reality of no-man's-land was that, under the dreadful conditions of trench warfare, with opposing armies living in close proximity for extended periods of time, troops often demonstrated a friendly spirit among each other and their wounded. It was not uncommon for battalion stretcher-bearers on both sides to divide no-man's-land between them, with each side handing over the other's wounded or informing the other of the position of its wounded to make rescue possible.[9]

Following a Turkish counterattack on Pope's Hill overlooking Anzac Cove in the Dardanelles campaign, hundreds of dead lay in "festering heaps" before the New Zealand and Australian trenches. An armistice granted on May 24, 1915, allowed both sides to bury their dead and collect their wounded. The areas in front of the parapets had become breeding grounds for blowflies and a nauseating source of discomfort to the defenders a few yards away. Wounded who had been lying in the open for three days were infested with maggots. In other areas, where opposing trenches were only a few yards apart, with murderous machine guns trained on the enemy dead to discourage burying parties, sanitary corpsmen resorted to grappling irons flung from the relative safety of trenches to drag the dead and decomposing bodies away for burial.[10]

Within the complications of battle, clearing the dead and wounded from the trenches and no-man's-land became a nightmarish spectacle. Following the first day's battle of the Somme on July 1, 1916, stretcher-bearers needed three days to clear the battle zone of more than fifty-seven thousand dead and wounded officers and men of the British army and nearly six thousand Germans. As many as ten thousand of the first day's wounded remained in the battle zone the following day, half of whom had not yet been accepted by a medical unit. Even after rescue, however, the wounded continued to suffer hardships. By the time surgeons could attend even minor wounds, the onset of gangrene necessitated lifesaving amputations to circumvent infection.[11]

EVACUATION STRATEGIES

On some days at the western front, the wounded numbered fewer than three hundred; on others, such as during the battle of the Marne, casualties soared above twenty thousand. During the first battle of the Marne, most of the Allied wounded arrived at hospitals without having been touched after the initial dressing. To complicate matters, the advancing Germans destroyed much of their transport; consequently, wounded arrived at field ambulances "in every imaginable condition." The lack of splints, first-aid dressings, shelter, and transportation took their inevitable toll. Wards filled with patients suffering from gas gangrene and tetanus as doctors scrambled for antitoxin, reverted to pre-aseptic surgical principles and practices, and initiated extensive clinical and laboratory research and experimentation.[12]

Military planners recognized that a successful evacuation depended on a number of variables, including the types of vehicles, the distance, the weather conditions, the roads, and the nature of the military operation. By dividing the evacuation area into zones, planners found it easier to understand the conceptual and practical implications of effective transport. In the first, or most advanced, zone, litter bearers transported the wounded; in the second—which included the regimental dressing stations and the hospital of evacuation (H.O.E.)—wagons, trench tramways, Decauville narrow-gauge field railways, and small, motor ambulances took over this responsibility. The Russian army Medical Corps used hardy Siberian ponies, while the French and Belgians sometimes used dogcarts. The next zone extended from the H.O.E. in the French service, the casualty clearing station in the British service, or the evacuation hospital in the American service to the base hospitals. This zone included road, rail, and water transportation. The final zone constituted the base section. When transport was available via canals and waterways, sanitary personnel used specially designed barges to transport patients with serious chest, head, or abdominal wounds. Each barge carried approximately thirty patients and conveyed them from the evacuation hospitals to base hospitals far in the rear. Hospital ships, painted white with a broad green band running from stem to stern and with red crosses on the sides and the funnel, accommodated from two hundred to three thousand wounded (plates 34, 35).[13]

At the outbreak of the war, ambulance companies among the Allied powers consisted of a captain, four first lieutenants, nine noncommissioned officers (two sergeants first class and seven sergeants), one cook, and sixty-nine privates first class. Twelve ambulances, three wagons, four pack mules, sixty draft animals, and thirteen mounts supported the personnel. Although Red Cross and civilian hospitals supplemented the medical needs of the military behind the war zone, no other organization bridged the critical area between the firing line and the hospital. Here, the ambulance company carried out its essential duties. All of the wounded, including the enemy, flowed through the ambulance company from battlefield to hospital.[14]

Ambulance-company officers assumed both organizational and professional responsibilities. Organization consisted of maintaining adequate supplies and equipment, ensuring the proper role and function of each man in the company, and managing the men, animals, and equipment in an orderly manner. Professional duties involved providing first aid for the sick and wounded, establishing appropriately administered dressing stations, and transporting evacuees in available conveyances from the battle line to the dressing station and from the dressing station to the field hospital. The efficiency and effectiveness of the medical evacuation system depended upon the proper understanding of these responsibilities.[15]

STRETCHER-BEARERS

The British supported two corps of stretcher-bearers: the Regimental Corps and the Royal Army Medical Corps (R.A.M.C.). The Regimental Corps, all volunteers, belonged to the battalion, wore its distinctive badge (white armlets initialed "S.B.," identifying them as stretcher-bearers), carried arms, and fought when necessary. In terms of numbers, there were 32 bearers per 1,000 men. The R.A.M.C. stretcher-bearers, on the other hand, were noncombatants, wore the distinctive Red Cross badge, and carried wounded from the regimental aid post to the nearest hospital. These bearers came under considerable shelling and suffered frequent casualties, unlike their predecessors in previous wars. Numbering around twenty thousand at the beginning of the war, they increased to about one hundred fifty thousand by war's end. During the course of the war, R.A.M.C. bearers administered to nine million cases.[16]

Regimental Corps bearers picked up wounded where they had fallen, rendered first aid, and took them from the front lines through narrow saps to the regimental aid posts located in sandbagged cupolas or cellars outside the field of machine-gun fire and managed by the battalion medical officer. During offensive operations, regimental bearers could not always keep pace with the casualties. With firepower concentrated at a few lines of trenches, the number of wounded multiplied enormously. At night, bearers cleared the no-man's-land under the flag of the Red Cross. Despite precautions, stretcher parties took hostile fire and, during major battles, sustained heavy casualties. In fact, it was common for stretcher-bearers to remove the white brassards, which made them easy targets for enemy marksmen.[17]

Transporting the wounded presented an arduous task for the stretcher-bearers, consuming nearly an hour for a round-trip of a thousand yards. Under continuous shelling, stretcher-bearers found it difficult to respond quickly to casualties and faced frequent exhaustion because of the increased distance between the front lines and the regimental aid posts and the ever-present mud, which clung to their feet as they carried the wounded.[18] For this reason, bearer companies remained as far forward as practicable to ensure speedy evacuation of the wounded. With luck, they could carry the wounded along evacuation trenches that were six to seven feet deep. On many occasions, however, because of the mud and the swampy nature of the soil, stretcher-bearers carried the wounded across open sections of the front before finding another trench. To be effective, they needed to study the terrain, identify nests where small groups of wounded could gather, assign areas of the battlefield to specific squads (to avoid covering the same ground twice), and be equipped with sufficient surgical dressings (plates 36–39). In severe engagements, when regimental personnel were unable to care for all of the wounded, the bearers provided first aid, as well as transportation.[19]

The topography of the front varied from sector to sector, forcing medical personnel to adapt to the terrain. In general, they organized their evacuation strategies into an elaborate system of relay stations that took advantage of entrenchments and every available means of effecting rapid evacuation.[20] Medical personnel had to have a thorough understanding of the successive lines of trenches during battle and know which were the "up" trenches and which were the "down." In other words, they could not block trenches by carrying wounded down when troops and ammunition were being taken up.[21]

Because the regulation stretcher proved too awkward for transport through the intricate network of trenches, bearers often improvised with a canvas sling suspended from a wooden pole or used an ordinary chair to carry the wounded. The stretcher carriage appealed to those bearers having to negotiate both rough and smooth terrain. Often, bearers improvised on the Ashford litter by fitting dragropes to its axles to increase their pace and reduce fatigue.[22] Bearers also adopted other systems, including carrying the wounded soldier in arms, by piggyback, by fireman's-carry, by pulling along the ground, by fore-and-aft carry, and by the two-hand seat and the four-hand seat. Stretchers included the regulation ambulance stretcher Mark II, the Rogers, and various improvised stretchers, using blankets, rifles, chairs, tunics, and assorted types of webbing. Although the Rogers stretcher predominated among the British regiments, the army permitted the use of other models, including the

Aubrey, Willis, Colt, Johnstone-Stirling, Goodacre, Graves, Langley-Jones, Butler, Welsh, Meek, Grant, and Robertson trench stretchers. Sanitary personnel also made use of the single-wheeled Blackham and Walker stretcher carriers, as well as the Hudlass and Smith, Victor, and Day carriers, which resembled wheelbarrows (plate 40). As armies settled into more permanent trench warfare, elaborate systems of evacuation evolved, including overhead trolleys that followed the network of trenches, a Barnton tramway over a narrow-gauge railway, and horse- or mule-drawn trucks over narrow-gauge railways. These railway or monorail systems (plate 41) carried wounded through the deep trenches to Decauville ambulance trains or tramcars. Light trolleys, constructed of wood and built on a four-wheeled bogie, carried two stretchers, one above the other, and ran along a narrow-gauge trench tramway. Pushed by two stretcher-bearers, the trolleys operated both in trenches and over open ground, usually in areas inaccessible to motor ambulances (plate 42). To assist in carrying the wounded, personnel often harnessed horses and mules to the trolleys.[23]

The Meerut Division first used a trench tramway in May 1915 during the battle of Festubert. Simply constructed of wooden rails and wooden trolleys, the tramway moved water and supplies to the regiments holding the fighting line and accommodated three recumbent cases on its return trip. By the end of 1915, four such tramways were in operation in the Meerut area alone. At the battle of Loos in September 1915, medical personnel improvised a similar system using the iron rails and trolleys found at nearby coal mines. During the later years of the war in France, the armies greatly expanded this system of evacuating wounded from the regimental aid posts. The Decauville railways, used principally to carry supplies and ammunition, also accommodated special or improvised ambulance trains (plate 43). The ambulance trains were fitted with stretchers, blankets, stoves, and they were staffed by R.A.M.C. personnel. During the battles of the Somme in 1916, these trains proved especially effective in evacuating the wounded.[24]

Other forms of transportation close to the battle line included Lewis gun carriages, modified to form stretcher carriers, and "mat stretchers," which personnel pulled through the trenches. In Gallipoli and Macedonia, the Sinai and southwest Africa, Russia, and elsewhere in the war theaters, armies used cacolets, attached to either side of a camel or mule (plate 44); the travois, constructed on the Greenleaf model used earlier by the United States in the western service; sand sledges and sleighs; stretchers carried crosswise and lengthwise on mules; and horse-drawn ambulance wagons (Mark V, Mark VI, and the Mark I [Light] ambulance), which carried from two to four recumbent, or six to twelve sitting, patients. Perhaps no problems of evacuation were more difficult than those experienced by stretcher-bearers on the beaches and gullies at Anzac Cove. Because of heavy rifle and machine-gun fire from the ridges, ambulance bearers faced enormous difficulty in removing the wounded, carrying them down narrow paths on improvised stretchers made of rifles and puttees, or glissading them down on sheets of oilcloth.[25]

The First Dressing

The nature of the first dressing, so it was commonly believed, determined the pathological course of a wound. In the Boer War, where the fighting occurred over largely unpopulated areas, where the climate remained sunny and dry, and where most wounds came from rifle bullets, wound complications were minimal. Indeed, the experiences of the war in South Africa and the Russo-Japanese War had been that, "in a large proportion of wounds, superficial or very casual chemical antisepsis, with immediate suture was not only permissible but desirable."[26] By contrast, the character of wounds and wound management in the Great War changed dramatically as shrapnel, trench mortars, bombs, and hand grenades created gashes and tears requiring major surgery. Shrapnel and compound fractures accounted for most of the wounds seen in hospitals. Bayonet wounds tended to be fatal, while those from hand grenades often resulted in eye injuries. As a further complication to wound management, soldiers lived in trenches and muddy terrain where microorganisms afflicted wounded and healthy alike. Working and sleeping in polluted soil and standing water, surrounded by garbage and human and animal feces, inundated by lice and fleas, and lacking proper hygiene and recreation, soldiers fell victim to all forms of infectious diseases.[27] Arthur Graham Butler, in *The Australian Army Medical Services in the War of 1914–1918* (1940), remarked that "the treatment of wounds in the field was vitiated by neglect of the fact that the infection was contained within the wound itself, so that for the most part paints of iodine or of picric alcohol were as whiting to a sepulchre, and repeated 'dressings' of little more use than were the antics and the offerings of the priests of Baal."[28]

Under these conditions, the first dressing given at the firing line, or at the *nid de blessés*, offered little protection against septic microorganisms. Cotton wool and absorbent, gauze dressings provided an ideal medium for bacteria. Substitutes, including muslin bags filled with pine sawdust, sterilized moss and peat moss, and crushed charcoal in gauze or in linen bags, offered little improvement. At best, the dressing stopped the bleeding, stabilizing the wound long enough for evacuation to a hospital where physicians and their attendants debrided the wound by surgically removing nonviable tissue and foreign matter, removing hematomas, and providing adequate drainage.[29]

During the early days of trench warfare, the British situated the regimental aid posts four hundred to fourteen hundred yards behind the front line, usually in a farmhouse or other convenient building, a reserve-trench dugout, or a shell hole. Later in the war, these stations took on the appearance of subterranean caves several stories deep, with pillars and crossbeams to prevent collapse during heavy shelling and canvas doors to protect against gas attacks. The regimental aid posts suffered heavily from shell fire and, during offensive operations, sometimes found themselves at the front line, or even beyond it. Nevertheless, there the field dressings were replaced with something more substantial, and amputations were performed for the most severe cases. There, too, the wounded received morphine injections, and the soldier's paybook was used to record the particulars of the wound and treatment. Regimental corpsmen then attached the information to the soldier's tunic to be read by subsequent medical personnel.[30]

Regimental surgeons rarely tended fractures, except to immobilize the limb for transportation, because of the difficulty in removing clothing or boots, the need to render the wound as clean as possible, and the potential danger of shock. Immobilizing the limb required various extemporaneous techniques at the battle line. Surgeons made splints out of rifles, sandbags, cardboard, trench implements, and anything else found in the vicinity of the battle area. Often, surgeons transformed the stretcher itself into a splint. Other transport splints included the Thomas arm splint, the Jones humerus traction splint, the Thomas traction leg splint, the long Liston splint, the Cabot posterior wire splint, the Jones crab or cock-up splint, and the ladder splint material.[31]

Following this initial aid, the wounded were moved to either first- or second-line divisional ambulances, which performed urgent operations and distributed patients by severity of their wounds. Situated in abandoned houses, the first-line ambulance offered only meager support, usually little more than a straw-covered floor on which to lie. The slightly wounded remained near the front, while those with moderate wounds traveled by sanitary train to the evacuation hospital of the army corps. The seriously wounded were moved to a nearby surgical ambulance. At the second-line ambulance, usually in a village with permanent buildings, surgeons treated wounds of the head, chest, and abdomen and performed more delicate operations. There, too, they worked to control hemorrhage and remove foreign bodies from the wounded area, performed debridement, adjusted fractures, and otherwise prepared patients for evacuation.[32]

Second-line ambulances held fifty to one hundred beds and faced overcrowding unless surgeons exercised good judgment in evacuating the wounded to a base hospital or in distributing to nearby ambulance hospitals those men too weak to travel. If treated efficiently, the wounded remained in the second-line ambulance less than a day before moving by horse-drawn wagon or motor vehicle to the *dépôt de éclopés*, sanitary train, canal boat, sanitary ship, base hospital, or other ambulance hospital. In France, good hospital facilities were within a twenty-four- to thirty-six-hour journey from the firing line.[33]

The casualty clearing station (C.C.S.), mobilized at the beginning of the war under the designation of "clearing hospital," was an English creation taking advantage of the availability of surgery at the front. Indeed, most of the surgical work performed during the war occurred at this station. "The proliferation of these miniature hospitals," wrote Denis Winter in *Death's Men: Soldiers of the Great War* (1978), "was due to the discovery that, if all dead and injured tissue was removed within thirty hours of damage, much sepsis and gangrene could be successfully dealt with."[34] Officially designated "casualty clearing stations" in January 1915 at the suggestion of Colonel Arthur Lee, they evacuated the field ambulances and forward patients to base hospitals. The C.C.S. quickly became the pivotal point in the collecting zone, the channel that connected the evacuating zone with the distributing zone. Located at an advanced base close to the division, it accommodated up to five hundred men at any one time. Originally, the C.C.S. had no transport of its own, relying instead upon empty supply wagons, motor-lorries, and horse transport belonging to other units. Before long, however, the C.C.S. took control of its own transportation. Located at such important junctions as Saint-Omer, Bailleul, Ypres, Poperinghe, Hazebrouck, and Béthune, these stations were near to both the fighting line and the critical railroad sidings for evacuation by train.[35]

Like the C.C.S., the French hospital of evacuation (H.O.E.) removed either temporarily or permanently the sick and wounded from the battle zone. As originally conceived in the 1910 French *Règlement*, the H.O.E. functioned as a temporary shelter for wounded soldiers being evacuated. However, the reality of the war imposed modifications unanticipated in the regulations. For one thing, the number of wounded was sometimes so high that medical personnel were faced with a dilemma: either hold severely wounded men without providing them with care, or evacuate them without regard to their precarious condition. Responding to this quandary, the French introduced a selection system, triage, designed to better classify those requiring immediate surgery, hospitalization, or evacuation. As the war took on a more stationary character, the H.O.E. tended to reflect that change by becoming little more than a hospital receiving wounded for specific treatment.[36]

Triage, from the French *trier*, meaning to pick, screen, choose, sort (out), or select, was first applied in 1727 to the English wool industry, where traders and manufacturers used the term to designate the separation or sorting of wool on the basis of its quality. A century later, the British had expanded the use of the term to apply to the coffee bean and the process of sorting out the fresh or finer-grade beans from those that were spoiled or of poorer quality. However, the military usage of the term *triage* originated with the French and meant both the place of sorting and the process of sorting, whereby patients were distributed to appropriate hospitals. In typical battle situations, the numbers of incoming wounded tended to overwhelm existing facilities and the treatment of already-consigned patients. On the assumption that the demand for medical services exceeded the available resources, decisions had to be made on the basis of priority, giving those in urgent need of medical attention greater priority over those with lesser wounds or those who were hopelessly wounded. Based on the premise that it was important to classify casualties for purposes of treatment and evacuation and that, in the circumstances of warfare, decisions had to be made giving preference to the good of the whole over the welfare of a particular individual, medical personnel sorted the wounded on the basis of those with slight injuries, those with wounds that required medical care but could be managed at an aid station or a divisional area before being returned to duty, those whose injuries demanded immediate attention, and those who were either dead or were wounded beyond hope.[37]

In response to the change in 1918 from a stationary war to one of movement, the French divided its H.O.E.s into hospitals of secondary (H.O.E.2) and primary (H.O.E.1) evacuation. The H.O.E.2 was designed for those whose surgical needs could be postponed and who could therefore be transported and treated at places more distant from the battle. In contrast, the H.O.E.1 received and triaged the sick, gassed, and wounded, classifying them into "very slight," "serious," and "nontransportable." It then treated and hospitalized the nonevacuable patients and prepared all other cases for evacuation or return to the front.[38]

Following its entry into the war in 1917, the U.S. Expeditionary Force First Infantry Division borrowed the triage idea from the Allies. Although several divisions eventually instituted triage at the dressing station, it was more commonly employed at the field hospital closest to the battle line. In trench warfare, a specifically designated hospital usually had the responsibility for triage; in open warfare, the field hospitals alternated the responsibility. However, the actual definition of triage varied among the American divisions. In some, the triage hospital "received all nontransportable patients whether sick, wounded, or gassed; in others it received the seriously wounded only; in yet others, as in the Thirty-sixth Division, this hospital retained no patients but was used solely as a distributing agency."[39]

THE GERMAN ARMY

First-aid stations did not differ substantially on either side of the battle line. The Austro-Hungarian army located its first-aid stations in trenches close to the firing line, connected by a communicating zigzag trench, or in a building or safe area one thousand to three thousand yards behind the line. Casualties remained in the trenches until nightfall, when they were removed to these stations. For artillery regiments, these first-aid stations were sometimes a half mile or more to the rear of the batteries, secure from the enemy's artillery. In the early part of the war, men wounded in cavalry patrols were carried on their own saddles or behind their comrades to medical stations in the rear of the encounters.[40]

Physicians seldom performed surgical work at the first-aid stations, preferring instead to dress wounds; apply splints; treat shock with adrenalin, cognac, or a solution of camphor; provide refreshment; give morphine to allay pain; fill out a transfer slip, which included the soldier's name and diagnosis (red tag for minor injuries, white for severe wounds); and prepare the wounded for evacuation. Sanitary personnel, assisted by bandsmen and other troops detailed for the purpose, cleared the first-aid stations using small wagons packed with straw to reduce the discomfort from heavy jolting.[41]

Sanitary personnel dressed wounds with tincture of iodine and injected each wounded soldier with 500 to 1,500 cc of tetanus antitoxin. They preferred starch bandages and wire splints to encourage discharge from the wound. The dressing stations kept those with abdominal injuries from four to six days and, except for ligation of arteries, performed no other operations. Men not transportable included those in shock or suffering from hemorrhage or abdominal wounds. Bedding consisted of straw placed over the floor and covered with blankets. Because of the distance to hospitals, patients often did not reach medical support for two or three days. This lapse allowed wounds to become infected, and where gas gangrene or tetanus developed, mortality rose.[42]

In the early period of trench warfare on the western front, injuries from explosive shells often turned to tetanus. In the region of Metz and Champagne, typhoid fever and dysentery made their appearance. On the eastern front, the German armies suffered major bouts of typhoid, dysentery, and then typhus fever, followed by cholera. To protect its interior lines, the German medical corps refused to evacuate contagious cases to base hospitals. Instead, the corps built eighteen "cleansing institutions," or delousing stations, on the eastern front and required all officers and enlisted men to pass through them on their way westward. On the western front, convalescents with dysentery and typhus were transported to Spa, Belgium, where they recuperated until ready to rejoin their regiments.[43]

Like the Allied armies, the Germans provided hospitals in the immediate rear of the battle zone to accommodate those too sick or gravely wounded to be evacuated. Because of the scarcity of motor ambulances, however, the German army relied primarily on animal-drawn wagons, railroads, and trolley tramways (plate 45) to connect their *lazaretts* with hospitals. The army also depended upon both regular- and narrow-gauge railroad service during the period of stationary warfare, including the use of auxiliary hospital trains consisting of empty freight coaches equipped with iron frames for litters. At the German frontier, the head of the Sanitary Transportation Commission took responsibility for further evacuation.[44]

Twenty-four thousand physicians served the German army during the course of the war, two-thirds of whom served in the field, the remainder in the home territory. Of this number, 562 died in battle, 763 died of disease, 2,149 were wounded, and 467 were listed as missing. In contrast, the Allies in the western theater commissioned 30,591 medical officers.[45]

GAS WARFARE

Notwithstanding the objections raised by Captain Alfred Thayer Mahan of the United States, the signatories to The Hague Peace Conference in 1899 agreed to abstain from the use of "asphyxiating or deleterious gases." The issue was again raised at The Hague Peace Conference in 1907, which reaffirmed the earlier statement and widened the definition to include the use of "poison or poisoned weapons" (Article 23). Clearly, the signatories understood the intent of the two conventions and, while the only force for the prohibition was a moral one, its significance could not be ignored. Thus, when the German High Command chose to use chlorine at Ypres, it breached these two conventions.[46]

At 5:00 P.M., April 22, 1915, following a fierce German bombardment, French Algerian riflemen and a French Zouave Division were engulfed in a yellowish green mist, which drifted across the level flats of Flanders in the vicinity of Poelkapelle, northeast of Ypres. Discharged from six thousand cylinders releasing nearly one hundred fifty tons, this cloud of chlorine gas, which lasted one and one-half hours, opened a new and grisly chapter in the war. The effects of the gas collapsed defenses, leaving a gap of nearly five miles between the French and British fronts. However, the surprise initiative halted when German troops ran into their own gas, and General Erich von Falkenhayn, who had provided no reserve troops, failed to exploit his success. The Allied defense fell entirely to Canadian troops who, when the Germans released a larger gas assault two days later in the early morning of April 24, held their ground, using the most primitive protection against the gas (urine-soaked masks, woolen socks padded with handfuls of damp earth and tied firmly over the mouth and nose, and hastily improvised masks consisting of a pad saturated with a solution of sodium carbonate and sodium hyposulfite). German hesitation and meteorological imprecision, together with British and Canadian resistance, halted this dramatic new technology. Six subsequent gas attacks during the second Ypres battle proved equally disappointing for the Germans, with one attack resulting in heavy German casualties because of a sudden change of wind. The tactical value of combining gas discharge and infantry attack continued to baffle military strategists, who increasingly saw gas as a weapon whose greatest strength lay not in its tactical superiority but rather in its role as a catalyst for confusion and low morale. However, the dangers of execution, even when weather conditions seemed suitable, remained problematic because the use of gas required extensive preparation behind the lines, and these preparations were increasingly obvious to airplane observation.[47]

Although the belligerents originally introduced gas as clouds generated from gas cylinders, they eventually delivered the gases in sixty-pound drums catapulted by Livens projectors (invented by British engineer Lieutenant Livens) or tube dischargers, four-inch Stokes mortars, and finally—with great accuracy at long range—by artillery shells and gas bombs. British retaliation for Ypres occurred on September 25, 1915, in the battle of Loos. Unfortunately for the British, the 150 tons of gas wafted back into their own trenches, poisoning many of the British soldiers. Unable to capitalize on its initial success, the British were eventually driven back to their original positions. On both sides of Loos, the gas-casualty rate was about 4.4 percent of all killed and wounded. Overall, gas casualties in the Great War numbered about 800,000: Russia, 295,000; France, 190,000; Great Britain, 181,000; Germany, 78,763; United States, 70,552; and Italy, 13,300.[48]

The gases included hydrocyanic acid and sulfur dioxide, nitric peroxide; the suffocant gases phosgene, diphosgene (Green Cross), chlorine, chloropicrin, stannic chloride, phenyl-carbylamine-chloride, cyanogen bromide, and dichlor-menthyl-ether; the vesicant gases lewisite (Dew of Death) and dichlor-ethyl-sulfide (British "mustard," French "Yperite," and German "Yellow Cross"); and the lachrimators, which included benzyl-bromide, bromacetone, acrolein, chloracetophenone, and brom-benzylcyanide. The two most widely used gases were phosgene and dichlor-ethyl-sulfide.[49]

Defensive measures against chlorine included mouth pads dampened with sodium thiosulfate to neutralize the acid gas, breathing through urine-soaked mouth pads or socks, respirators made of waterproof pouches that held cotton waste dampened with thiosulfate, and even breathing through loosely packed earth. Later, when phosgene, chloropicrin, and diphosgene were used, scientists introduced filters consisting of pumice treated with potash and hexamine, potassium carbonate, and charcoal. Actually, the number of different alkalies tested included tiosulfate, sodium ricinoleate, sodium sulfanilate, sodium phenate, and hexamine. The English wore masks known as the black veiling respirator, the hypo helmet, the P and PH helmets, and the box respirator. The French had their M-2 mask; the Tissot mask used principally by artillerymen, stretcher-bearers, and those required to work with greater efficiency; and the A.R.S. mask (*appareil respiratoire spécial*), which allowed the soldier to breathe through a small metal drum filled with absorbent cotton, charcoal, soda lime, and zinc oxide moistened with glycerin.[50]

Although the pathology of gassing remained uncertain through most of 1915, it became clear to medical personnel that the severity of the symptoms depended upon the duration of exposure and the concentration of gas breathed by the troops. Immediate medical evacuation and fresh air were two obvious remedies for gassed victims. Unfortunately, this was no easy task since the casualty clearing stations and motor ambulances were still in their early forms of organizational development. Moreover, unacquainted with the different stages of gassing, the differences in effects among the types of gases, and the forms of treatment, medical personnel found themselves at a loss for providing relief. For many, the plight of gas victims became horribly demoralizing as they watched men drown in their own body fluids. As one nurse commented,

> Gas cases are terrible. They cannot breathe lying down or sitting up. They just struggle for breath, but nothing can be done. Their lungs are gone— literally burnt out. Some have their eyes and faces entirely eaten away by gas and their bodies covered with first-degree burns. We must try to relieve

them by pouring oil on them. They cannot be bandaged or touched. We cover them with a tent of propped-up sheets. Gas burns must be agonizing because usually the other cases do not complain even with the worst wounds but gas cases are invariably beyond endurance and they cannot help crying out. One boy today, screaming to die, the entire top layer of his skin burnt from face and body. I gave him an injection of morphine. He was wheeled out just before I came off duty. Where will it end?[51]

The suffocant gases were pulmonary irritants, which created acute inflammation of the lungs, destruction of the alveolar epithelium, bursting of air vesicles, emphysema, and heart failure. Because chlorine is heavier than air, it settled in shell holes and trenches, where it quickly overcame those who inhaled it in any quantity. The irritation caused by the gas created intense inflammation of the bronchi-pulmonary.[52]

Mustard gas (dichlor-ethyl-sulfide), which the Germans introduced July 12–13, 1917, during the third Ypres battle, caused a wholly different set of symptoms. More toxic than phosgene and vaporizing very slowly, it remained on the ground for days, even weeks, after an attack and produced nearly eight times the number of casualties as other gases. Unlike other gases, it had very little immediate effect on the respiratory system or the eyes, and soldiers often came in contact with it unknowingly. Irritation did not develop until three to twelve hours after exposure. Thus, armies employed it as a neutralizing gas rather than as a surprise gas, particularly in valleys and woods, which tended to retain the gas for longer periods of time. Armies also employed the gas against artillery emplacements, against support and reserve positions, and against communicating trenches and roads.[53]

The effects of mustard and other vesicant gases included progressive conjunctivitis, rapidly developing blisters, bronchitis, inflammation of the lungs, and long-term disability. Treatment included mobile bathing units attached to the collecting station; fresh clothing; and sodium bicarbonate solution for the eyes, nose, and throat; intravenous injections of gum glucose solution; the occasional use of venesection (500 to 750 cc) in cyanotic cases; and oxygen and intravenous injections of caffeine sodium benzoate.[54]

Mustard gas proved especially difficult to detect and, as already stated, infantry discovered that the gas remained dangerous for days and even weeks after a shelling, clinging to clothes, weapons, and other materials. Even treating the impact areas with bleaching powder did not always solve the problems encountered when soldiers accidentally touched walls, machinery, and other items covered by the gas. Because of production problems, the French did not begin using mustard gas until June 1918, and the British were delayed until September of the same year.[55] According to Edward S. Farrow in *Gas Warfare* (1920),

> The best protection against mustard gas is evacuation of all ground infected by it, if the tactical situation permits, and alternative positions should be prepared or selected in advance. If a zone has been evacuated after a mustard gas bombardment, sentries should be posted on all roads and paths entering this zone to warn troops away from it and to prevent their entering. Sentries should also be posted in front of contaminated dugouts in a zone otherwise free from mustard gas. If not possible to evacuate, frequent reliefs, or protection of troops as far as possible in gasproof dugouts will alone prevent numerous casualties, as mustard gas will outlast the staying power of troops wearing the respirator. In connection with the use of gasproof dugouts, it should be noted that men entering such dugouts have gassed the occupants by the gas which they have brought in on their clothes and, therefore, all outer clothing should be removed in the entrance to the dugout and soles of shoes treated with chloride of lime. A scraper, water, and box of chloride of lime should be kept near the entrance to each dugout. The shoes are first dipped into the water, then thoroughly rubbed in the lime, and finally washed off in the water. This precaution, if followed by thorough washing of the body, will be very effective in preventing burns.[56]

Litter bearers and ambulance personnel faced difficult problems in evacuating the wounded and decontaminating their supplies, food, clothes, and motor transportation from mustard gas (plate 46). Regimental aid posts, dressing stations or field ambulances, and casualty clearing stations were forced to adjust quickly. The British evacuated all gas cases as quickly as possible to the regimental aid posts, where personnel washed the victims and gave them clean clothes, oxygen, and other treatment. From there, the gas victims moved to the C.C.S. for classification, segregation, additional oxygen treatment, and eventual evacuation. The French established for each corps disinfectant stations that included showers, oxygen equipment, and trained medical staff. The Germans introduced special centers or stations for gas cases, while the Americans created separate gas hospitals for treatment and convalescence. Understandably, the creation of separate facilities for gas victims resulted in severe demands being placed on human and material resources. Nevertheless, the morale problems created by gas warfare necessitated the segregation of gas victims.[57]

6

Trials of Evacuation

Although certain armchair critics doubted the reliability of motorized transport and persisted in advocating animal-drawn conveyances, motor vehicles quickly demonstrated their value in the movement of men, supplies, and ammunition in the Great War. The British Royal Expeditionary Force, for example, began with 950 lorries and 250 motorcars; by armistice, it had 33,500 lorries, 1,400 tractors, 13,800 motorcars, and thousands of motorcycles in use. Armies also achieved decisive tactical advantages with requisitioned cars and buses with which they moved reinforcements into the field. Moreover, auxiliary support, in the form of searchlights, field kitchens, wireless stations, and repair shops, all benefited from the internal-combustion engine. Army medical units established motor hospitals with antiseptic operating rooms fitted with hot and cold water. The French army even maintained a mobile X-ray machine, with instruments operated by electricity, and "flying bacteriological laboratories" that, equipped with scientific apparatus, moved about the front, identifying typhoid and dysentery in the field.[1] While the airplane and dirigible seemed to catch the eye of the press, the motorcar and -truck demonstrated broad capability for replenishing food and ammunition supplies and for overall transportation and ambulance support. Some military observers, in fact, characterized the conflict not as the "Great War" but as the "Automobile War." Notwithstanding this laudatory recognition, horse-drawn ambulances still predominated for all belligerents.[2]

THE AUTOMOBILE WAR

Equipping British field ambulances with motor vehicles received official approval in November 1914. This decision did not come without a baptism of fire, for during the battle of Mons, August 22–23, 1914, British efforts to clear the wounded to dressing stations and to railway depots broke down completely. There simply were not enough horsed ambulance wagons, empty supply lorries, or organized ambulance trains. During this engagement, medical personnel sought permission to improvise ambulance wagons on the chassis of local taxicabs. Although refused by the inspector general of communications, the effort signaled the eventual introduction of motorized ambulance cars to the British expeditionary force in France and heralded the subsequent formation of motor-ambulance convoys for the Royal Army Medical Corps. By September, the British had several motor ambulances, which had been donated by the French; and by November 1914, the first field ambulances were equipped with motor vehicles.[3]

Had motorized transport been available to the British after Mons and Le Cateau (August 26), the number of wounded taken prisoner would have been negligible. However, not until the first battle of Ypres (October 30 to November 24) did armies recognize the full impact of motorized support. There, sanitary personnel moved patients quickly to clearing stations, thereby preventing the wounded from falling into enemy hands. Ironically, the motorized ambulance circumvented the intent of the Geneva Convention: the army with the most effective ambulance system collected more wounded, including those belonging to the enemy, sometimes tempting armies to interdict the efforts of the enemy's Red Cross by force.[4]

In the early months of the war, ambulance units evacuated the wounded in returning supply convoys. This method, which resulted in part from poor planning, met with abject failure, something that Lord Douglas Haig had predicted as early as 1913.[5] Soon afterward, General Headquarters decided to form motor-ambulance convoys and equip them with fifty ambulance cars. To achieve this, sanitary personnel accepted motorcars of all makes and designs for ambulance support, and volunteers (using their own or borrowed touring cars) rendered valuable assistance to the armies on the western front. The cars included the Austen, Buick, Clement-Talbot, Crossley, Daimler, Dennis, Fiat, Ford, Mors, Napier, Panhard, Renault, Rolls Royce, Sheffield Simplex, Siddeley Deasy, Straker-Squire, Studebaker, Denain, Vauxhall, Sunbeam, Vulcan, and Wolsley. Of those, the Daimler, Sunbeam, Fiat, Wolsley, Austen, and Ford were the most reliable. The French also requisitioned Paris Renault taxis to rush men and supplies to the Marne, as well as to carry wounded back from the front. During active operations, the ambulances were supported by motortrucks, omnibuses, and charabancs. The French supplemented these with motorcycles with a sidecar attachment designed to carry a single stretcher. Medical support units objected to motor-lorries as a "fool's paradise," for they were invariably unclean and uncomfortable. In emergencies, however, even the motor-lorries were preferable to horse-drawn wagons; a few gallons of petrol and one driver did the work of two men, four horses, and fodder.[6]

Faced with unprecedented numbers of casualties, the British Red Cross Society, the St. John Ambulance Brigade, medical journals, and popular magazines appealed for donations of private automobiles. Requests urged individuals, especially "such folk as keep a stud of motor carriages," to donate their cars to the British Red Cross Society or to the St. John Ambulance Brigade for use at the front or behind the line. In patriotic response, members of the Royal Automobile Club and the Automobile Association of Great Britain generously offered their vehicles. The British Red Cross Society assumed no responsibility for deterioration or loss of property; owners understood that they loaned their vehicles unconditionally, accepting any damage incurred.[7] Through the Automobile Association of Great Britain, members lent more than nineteen thousand motorcars and -cycles to transport wounded from ports and railheads to designated hospitals and to remove wounded from London hospitals to convalescent centers scattered across the nation. The obvious advantage of the light automobile was its speed and maneuverability in railway yards and hospital compounds.[8]

Patriotic and voluntary aid societies were active in assisting all of the belligerent nations, and New Zealand was no exception. In early August 1914, the New Zealand War Contingent Association formed to provide benevolent support for the war effort. In October of the same year, the dominion government ordered fourteen motor ambulances from England, of which ten were paid for by individuals or voluntary aid societies. The New Zealand branch of the British Red Cross stocked each ambulance with extra medical stores and dressings. Other agencies—the Red

Cross, the St. John's Ambulance Brigade, the Young Men's Christian Association (Y.M.C.A.), and the Salvation Army—contributed gifts, money, and personnel for service to the sick and wounded.[9]

The motor ambulance required one-tenth the storage space of a mule and saved one-third to one-half the transportation time. Although motor vehicles suffered chronic tire problems, the war became a proving ground, demonstrating their efficiency and dependability beyond all expectations. As one enthusiastic observer noted, "Hot weather is no bar to speed. No harnessing is needed for starting and no feeding, unharnessing and bedding has to be done at night when the soldier is tired out. The automobile stands without hitching, and it hauls other vehicles, and is more dependable and there is an evener pull. It is under absolute control of the driver and instant control of the brake. The cost of maintenance is one-fourth that required of mules. There is no fatigue to the motor."[10] This was in sharp contrast to the support systems required for horses and mules.

On all fronts, at any one time, horses and mules totaled over a million, with 436,000 in France alone. Like soldiers, horses and mules were susceptible to disease, as well as to disabling conditions caused by shrapnel, bombs, gas poisoning, and other complications. Their maintenance, care, segregation, and disposal required extensive planning, organization, and manpower. During offensive operations, the wastage of animals from exhaustion and debility reached unprecedented heights, not only on the western front but in mounted operations in Egypt and Palestine, the advance to Baghdad, winter operations on the Salonika front (1915), and the final stages of operations in southwest Africa. As with the evacuation of wounded soldiers, the circumstances of war required an extensive ambulance system for sick and injured animals, with dressing stations situated between the firing line and the mobile veterinary section. Successful evacuation along the lines of communication included the use of advanced collecting posts, veterinary evacuating stations, veterinary hospitals, and convalescent horse depots. The methods of transport included horse-drawn ambulances, motor-driven horse ambulances, sick-horse trains, and barges. The British Royal Army Veterinary Service in France alone numbered 651 officers and fifteen thousand other men.[11]

Before motorized ambulances came into general use, distances to vital railheads became a matter of horse and human endurance. Transport from field ambulances to the advance base required massive efforts, much of which had to be accomplished at night to avoid shelling. The new conditions brought on by the motorcar, combined with the close network of railroads and the proximity of towns and villages, meant that doctors and surgeons could usually provide adequate medical support within a reasonable time from the moment the soldier was wounded. Despite the obvious benefits of motor transport, the military wisely chose to retain horse-drawn ambulances, demonstrating their usefulness during the Somme offensive in 1916, where they transported wounded from areas with no roads or where roads were impassable because of artillery fire or mud. As late as 1918, gasoline shortages made it necessary to employ horsed ambulance wagons where possible.[12]

With increased artillery range, field hospitals moved further to the rear of the firing line, necessitating a more efficient transport vehicle and evacuation system. Horses drawing ambulances were simply unable to endure the distances imposed by the new conditions and still deliver wounded to hospital bases within a reasonable time. The motor ambulance overcame these difficulties by providing ready access to hospitals and supplies, even when distances of forty miles or more separated division and railhead. Motor ambulances offered easier loading and unloading of stretchers, smoother transportation, protection from the elements, and, most importantly, quick response. They also reduced the amount of support required of horses and decreased as well the distance at which the headquarters of the field ambulance operated behind the firing line. Ten miles became the approximate distance between the headquarters of the ambulance and the front. Overall, motor ambulances resulted in a safer and more rapid evacuation of wounded and clearly counteracted the "long sweep of modern artillery and aircraft which otherwise would have made the transference of wounded to a place where they could be attended to in rest and quiet a very serious matter."[13]

Typically, the motorized ambulance convoy transported the sick and wounded from the dressing stations to the casualty clearing station (C.C.S.). During battle, the convoy cars carried only stretcher cases and those seriously injured who could sit; ambulatory wounded moved by motor-lorries and horsed ambulances. Occasionally, sanitary personnel held motor convoys in reserve to evacuate cases from one C.C.S. to another further back when ambulance trains were unavailable. Because time and weight factored so heavily in a successful evacuation, ambulance companies deliberately limited their equipment to a few essential articles (i.e., blankets, extra splints and dressings, bandages, and drinking water) to assist in the comfort of patients. Additional items simply took up space and created potential weight problems in the muddy terrain of the war zone.[14]

From their early experiences, the military quickly learned the benefits of light-car ambulances, the inappropriateness of battery-operated vehicles, the emergencies that sometimes necessitated carrying eight to ten patients in space provided for four, the mechanical difficulties of high-geared pleasure cars, the weight limits of springs, the benefits of double rear wheels, the impediments of wind resistance, and the need for sufficient ground clearance and a short wheelbase. Ambulance drivers preferred lower-geared vehicles for mud and rough terrain, extralarge wheels to ensure comfort for the wounded, and a low center of gravity for the chassis.[15]

With so many private cars serving as ambulance carriers, differences in chassis, motor, wheel size, gears, speed, and transmission drive meant that no single standard predominated. In response to difficulties resulting from this lack of standardization, the British Red Cross Society requested that the *Cooper's Vehicle Journal*, the official journal of the coach-building industry, design an ambulance body that would fit various types of chassis. The experiences at the front clearly demonstrated the need for revisions in motorized ambulance construction. The coach industry, recognizing the merits of the idea, built ambulance bodies for the British Red Cross Society in conjunction with several motor manufacturers. By 1915, Napiers and Vauxhalls came equipped with ambulance bodies meeting these new specifications, particularly the lack of overhang, a longer wheelbase, and a lower center of gravity.[16]

Depending on their size and design, motor ambulances carried two, four, or six recumbent cases and from four to eight sitting (plates 47, 48). Ambulances usually received the stretcher from behind or, as with the Austrian and French models, from the side. Depending also upon the particular design, personnel placed stretchers directly on the floor of the ambulance in the Ford, on rails in the Daimler, or on rigid arms in the Denain. One troublesome issue was whether litters should fit into trays or hang from straps. Experience indicated that elaborate methods of sling suspension delayed loading time and complicated the speedy evacuation of the wounded.[17]

Given the structural drawbacks of existing motorcars, some builders chose to construct ambulance trailers rather than attempt to convert motorcars. Built at minor cost, the trailer attached to the rear of the motorcar and used pneumatic tires for a smoother ride. The same ingenuity that went into building ambulance trailers applied to motorcycles and their sidecars. F. W. Barnes, of the Zenith Company in London, designed and patented a motorcycle constructed with one forward wheel and two in the rear to accommodate both the driver and a sidecar.[18]

Two types of ambulance bodies emerged out of the war experience. The first was the *American ambulance type*, built on a Ford chassis. Although it initially accommodated four stretchers, weight problems forced a change to a three-stretcher car. Other alterations occurred as well, including the use of larger tires and an additional leaf in the rear spring. The Ford had the advantage of lightness, good ground clearance, adequate engine power, and easy movement through mud and fields without becoming stuck. Constructed of wood and canvas and designed for economy of space, it became known as a "soapbox body." Despite its maneuverability, drivers found themselves continually working on some mechanical problem, whether a bent axle, leaky radiator, or worn-out bearings.[19]

Ford ambulance bodies were constructed in France, even after America's entry into the war. An assembly and revision plant was established on Rue de St. Ouen, Paris. There, chassis shipped from base ports in the United States were put together and fitted with bodies furnished by French manufacturers. Here, too, mechanics overhauled worn-out motor ambulances, touring cars, and trucks, making them again fit for service. Because of its short wheelbase, the Ford body projected out beyond the rear wheels. Despite this amusing appearance, the Ford maneuvered well and could turn on a short radius. With a reinforcing rear spring, the Ford rode high off the ground and gained a reputation for traveling over rough roads more easily than could other motorized ambulances. Although the Ford was designed for three lying or five sitting cases, it was not unusual for seven or eight wounded to be carried in times of emergency. On better roads to the rear of the dressing stations, however, ambulance personnel preferred the more comfortable General Motors ambulances.[20]

During the battle of Verdun in 1916, the Ford ambulance earned the respect of the sanitary corps and the fighting regiments. According to the London *Daily Telegraph*,

> For fully three months, until railways could be built, France kept up this endless chain of four thousand autos, two thousand moving up one side of the roadway from Bar-le-Duc and the other two thousand moved on the opposite side from Verdun. . . . Hundreds of lives would have been lost had it not been for the sections of the American Field Service stationed at Verdun. Equipped with small, light, speedy cars, capable of going almost anywhere and everywhere that the heavy French auto-ambulances could not go, the "rush" surgical cases were given to these American drivers. They were not given a place in the endless chain, but were allowed to dart into the intervening space of sixty feet maintained between the cars, and then make their way forward as best they could. When an open field offered, they left the road entirely, and, driving across, would come back into line when they could go no farther and await another chance for getting ahead. They were able to bring the wounded down from Verdun often twice as fast as those who came in the regular ambulances, and always without ever committing the one

great error upon which the life of France depended, the tying up for a single instant of the endless chain of the four thousand automobiles of Verdun.[21]

The Allies welcomed American ambulances, particularly the Ford. Nicknamed "the goat" by the French soldiers in Alsace and the "Chinese Rolls Royce" and "mechanical flea" by the British, the Ford showed its prowess in climbing hills, in off-road mobility, and in muddy terrain. With its low profile, the Ford could move close to the firing line without attracting the enemy's fire.[22] The following poem typified the folklore surrounding the Ford ambulance and the status it held among American and Allied army personnel.

HUNKA TIN

You may talk about your voitures
As you're sittin' round your quarters,
But when it comes to bringin' blessés in,
Take a little tip from me,
Let those heavy motors be:
Pin your faith on Henry Ford's old
      Hunka Tin.

I've been round this war
Six, seven months or more,
It doesn't matter when it begin;
And I've seen a car or so,
But the best one that I know
Is that ridiculed old junk heap, Hunka Tin.
Give her essence and de l'eau,
Crank her up and let her go,
You back-firin', spark-plug foulin'
      Hunka Tin.

The paint is not so good,
And no doubt you'll find the hood
Will rattle like a boiler shop en route;
The cooler's sure to boil
And perhaps she's leakin' oil,
And oftentime the horn declines to toot;
But when the night is black,
And there's blessés to take back,
And they hardly give you time to take a smoke,
It's mighty good to feel,
As you're sittin' at the wheel,
She'll be runnin' when the bigger cars are broke.

Oh, it's Tin, Tin, Tin!
If it happens there's a ditch you've skidded in,
Don't be worried, but just shout
Till some Poilu boosts you out,
And you're glad she's not so heavy,
      Hunka Tin.

After all the wars are past
And we're taken home at last,
To our reward of which the preacher sings;
When these ukelele sharps
Will be strummin' golden harps
And the avions all have regular wings;
When the Kaiser is in hell
With the furnace drawin' well,
Payin' for his million different kinds of sin;
If they're runnin' short of coal,
Show me how to reach the hole,
And I'll dump a few loads down with
      Hunka Tin.

Yes, Tin, Tin, Tin!
You exasperatin' puzzle, Hunka Tin.
I've abused you and I've flayed you,
But, by Henry Ford that made you,
You are better than the Big Uns,
      Hunka Tin.[23]

The second style of motor ambulance, known as the *French army type Kellner*, fitted many different makes and powers of chassis, although its best performance came from those with twelve to fifteen horsepower rather than the high-powered luxury cars. Its design developed more slowly than had the Ford's, evolving through several stages, the first being the "angle-iron canvas." Although the primitive construction of the canvas design gave little protection to the wounded during transportation, the Kellner did accommodate six stretchers attached to the roof by spring-supported leather hangers. Canvas covered the roof, front, and sides, and the rear had a canvas curtain to permit easy loading.[24]

Over the course of the war, innovations in the Kellner included a fixed roof over the driver; windows; room for five, rather than six, stretcher cases; and a longer body for easier loading and unloading. The four upper stretchers were suspended from leather hangers. In addition, the Kellner ambulance could seat eight patients lengthwise along the side, bringing the total capacity to five stretcher cases and eight seated, or two stretcher cases and fourteen seated. Experience, however, showed that floor stretchers were more comfortable than those suspended from the roof or sides and that the rear canvas curtains did little to keep out winter cold and summer dust.[25]

Later changes in the Kellner design included a hood over the driver's seat that folded back for better vision when driving without lights. Wooden shutters replaced the canvas curtains in the rear. The upper stretchers now rested on slides rather than on hangers; this change improved the loading time and made the ride more comfortable. Finally, the new design included storage boxes on each side of the car for reserve gasoline, tools, and personal baggage.[26]

By the end of the war, most motor ambulances were designed to withstand heavy field service, with three-ply wood construction; heavy, waterproof material; hard oak or thick linoleum flooring; celluloid roll-up screens, in place of glass windows or side panes; easy-to-reach brake and clutch pedals; and a wide wheelbase. Despite these changes, ambulance drivers and attendants continually faced the problem of maintaining sufficient warmth for those suffering shock or hemorrhage. Most early ambulances provided only a lamp for warmth; later models offered radiating heat by electrical heating or transferred engine exhaust or radiator water through pipes into the interior. As a rule, however, sanitary corpsmen faced chronic problems with the cold and drafts despite efforts to use curtains, hinged doors, and other arrangements.

AMERICAN VOLUNTEERS

United States' relief activities originated with Americans living in Paris years before the war who established an American hospital at Neuilly-sur-Seine. The hospital eventually became a rallying point for American residents, students, and travelers visiting or living in Paris at the opening of the war. The American relief effort in France began with the collection of motorcars and evolved quickly into evacuating wounded soldiers as the battle closed in on Paris. The efforts begun by this hospital were later supplemented by volunteers and funds from private citizens and American relief organizations.[27]

At first, the French army refused to permit neutrals, including Americans, to enter the war zone. Not until April 1915, as a result of the efforts of Inspector of the Field Service A. Piatt Andrew, did the French General Headquarters authorize volunteer ambulance sections in the French army. Formerly an assistant professor of economics at Harvard University and later assistant secretary of the United States Treasury Department, Andrew threw himself into the war effort by assembling three sections of cars and volunteer drivers to assist the French. The agreement reached between Andrew and the French signified direct cooperation among American volunteers and the French army in the advanced zone and actually incorporated the volunteer units within and under the direct authority of the French army, marking the beginning of the American Field Service, or the American Ambulance Field Service as it was originally called. Numbering approximately two thousand, these volunteers became a recognized part of every battle along the French front. The service began with a gift of ten Ford ambulances with bodies made from packing boxes; as donations multiplied, volunteer squads, consisting of five cars each, organized to offer service with the armies.[28]

Initially, the French sent a squad of ten American ambulances to the Vosges, where they formed an independent sanitary section and took over a sector on the front in Alsace. The success of this section led to the establishment of other units and, by the end of April, the American Ambulance Field Service had become a reality, comprising three sections of twenty ambulances each. *Section Sanitaire Américain No. 1* was at Dunkirk, *Section Sanitaire Américain No. 2* moved to Lorraine, and *Section Sanitaire Américain No. 3* located at the Vosges. *Section No. 1* eventually moved to Belgium at Coxyde, Nieuport, Poperinghe, Elverdinghe, Crombec, and elsewhere on the front. *Sections Nos. 2* and *3* worked the *postes de secours* (aid stations) on the line and became independently responsible for their respective service areas. By 1916, the Field Service of 349 volunteers included eighty-nine men from Harvard, twenty-six from Yale University, twenty-three from Princeton University, eight from the University of Michigan, four from the University of Virginia, eighteen Rhodes scholars from Oxford University, and men from thirty additional colleges and universities (plate 49). By January 1917, Andrew boasted more than two hundred cars driven by American volunteers grouped into sections of the French army; and by the time the United States entered the war, the ambulance sections of the American Field Service had grown to thirty-four, while the Red Cross had twelve sections in operation. Although most sections operated along the French front, two were sent to the Balkans. There, they worked with French troops in northern Greece, Serbia, and Albania.[29]

American university students who served in France, Belgium, and the Near East included Richard Norton, son of Charles Eliot Norton. Formerly director of the American School of Classical Studies in Rome, Richard Norton organized the American Volunteer Motor-Ambulance Corps and, by October 1914, ten of his ambulances were working with the British Red Cross and the St. John Ambulance Brigade. Later, the corps became associated with the American Red Cross and worked under the direct control of the French Eleventh Army Corps. Described by Norton as "wanderers searching for work," the corps found themselves immediately put into medical evacuation work and, by the end of 1915, had carried some twenty-eight thousand cases. By the time America entered the war, Norton had more than one hundred ambulances under his charge on the western front.[30]

The young ambulance drivers were volunteers (similar in status to the American aviators of the Lafayette Escadrille), typically from prominent American families, and representing nearly every region of the country. They included Malcolm Cowley, John Dos Passos, Ernest Hemingway, Julian Green, William Seabrook, e. e. cummings, Slater Brown, Harry Crosby, Sidney Howard, Louis Bromfield, Robert Hillyer, and Dashiell Hammett.[31] Their reasons for joining the Field Service were many; some showed genuine idealistic motives, while others joined for the excitement. One driver admitted he had volunteered "with the object of seeing war at firsthand and of getting some excitement, as well as being of some service." For Julien H. Bryan, whose previous job had been with the New York Central Railroad, the opportunity to become a volunteer represented an escape from boredom.[32] According to Edwin Wilson Morse, in *The Vanguard of American Volunteers in the Fighting Lines and in Humanitarian Service*, "The old law of noblesse oblige pointed the way to duty unerringly, and [the young men] followed it unhesitatingly." By the time of America's declaration of war in April 1917, some 533 graduates and undergraduates of Harvard alone found service functions in Europe—from actual fighting to hospital and ambulance work.[33]

This aspect of American volunteerism has been richly documented in personal reminiscences, diaries, and novels. The diaries and stories published by the American Ambulance Field Service in its *Friends of France* (1916) recounts in graphic detail the dangers faced by them through the course of the war.

> To go from this place to the sorting-point behind the lines to which the wounded are taken is the worst run we have. It means almost wondering if your car will make the grades, if you acted properly in letting yourself be persuaded to take three wounded instead of the specified two. It means coming upon comrades *en panne* and lending a hand or hurrying on with the distress signal, stopping to pour water into your boiling radiator, halting to pass convoys, arguments, decisions, "noms-de-Dieu," backing into a wider place, wheels that nearly go over the edge, pot-bellied munition-wagons that scrape off your side boxes, getting into a ditch and having to be pulled

out by mules or pushed out by men. It is a journey fraught with worry, for there is always the danger of delay when delay may mean death and is sure to mean suffering for the wounded in your car. And sometimes when, with bad cases aboard, you are stuck and can't get out until somebody turns up to help you, it is unbearable to stay near your car and hear their pitiful groans.[34]

The officers and personnel of an American volunteer sanitary section consisted of a commanding officer (second lieutenant of the French army), bookkeeper (sergeant of the French army), American officers under the command of a French lieutenant, and other personnel who included several American mechanics. The American volunteers usually enlisted for six months. The drivers and assistant drivers received the same pay and rations as the French soldiers—about five cents per day, an amount usually augmented by the American relief organizations that financed the sections. Only the mechanics received regular wages funded by the sponsoring organizations. The French army provided minor maintenance, gasoline, and tires, while the sponsor financed more extensive repairs in shops established at Kellner's in Billancourt.[35]

Banker Herman Harjes financed one contingent of American volunteers known as the *Harjes Ambulance Corps*. Along with the Norton unit with which it was later consolidated under the auspices of the American Red Cross, the Harjes Ambulance Corps was furnished with funds for an ambulance section, including salaries for a cook and two mechanics and for food, uniforms, and equipment. The ambulances consisted of Packards, Renaults, Panhards, Motoblocs, and Bertiets. With the exception of the Packards, the cars were nearly unusable, the oldest having been built in 1907.[36]

Immediate problems facing the ambulance sections stemmed from the diversity of contributed motorcars, their need for further construction before becoming usable to the army, and the lack of interchangeable spare parts. At one time, as many as 352 different forms of motorized transport were used by the belligerent powers, including 281,000 different types of spare parts.[37] As a result, the Field Service decided early in the war not to accept gifts of miscellaneous cars; instead, it chose the Ford motorcar as its standard, importing some twelve hundred chassis into France (plate 50). As A. Piatt Andrew noted, however, Henry Ford offered little assistance in this endeavor. Because of the automaker's "peculiar ideas of philanthropy" and his opposition to war activities of any type, "we could obtain not even the favor of wholesale rates in the purchase of cars and parts, and for every Ford car and for every Ford part imported from America, in those difficult days before America came into the war, we were obliged to pay, not the dealer's price, but the full market price charged to ordinary retail buyers."[38] Each ambulance section had attached to it twenty Ford ambulances, two in reserve, a Ford staff car, a light repair car designed to carry spare parts, a two-ton repair truck, a two-ton truck designed to carry fifteen to twenty sitting cases, a kitchen trailer, and three tents.[39]

At the time the United States officially entered the war, the American Field Service counted twelve hundred volunteers within the French army. The high regard in which the French held the Field Service was evident in an appeal to the American government in the spring of 1917 that, in the event of an American declaration of war, the United States should "reloan" the Field Service to France so that it could continue functioning as before, only under American control. After declaring war, the United States provided an additional five thousand light ambulances and six thousand enlisted men to support the Field Service. In this way, the cars and their support teams continued to serve the French without interruption. A similar relationship existed between the U.S. Army Ambulance Service and the Italian army. Although Marshal Joseph-Jacques-Césaire Joffre requested fifty ambulance sections in addition to the thirty-seven sections organized by the American Red Cross, only about twenty-five were actually put into operation by the U.S. Army Ambulance Service. Unlike animal-drawn ambulances supplied by the Quartermaster Corps, the procurement of motor ambulances became the direct responsibility of the Medical Department for the greater part of the war. In all, the United States Army shipped 3,070 General Motors ambulances and 3,805 Ford ambulances to France and Italy for the war effort.[40]

In typical battle situations, animal-drawn ambulance companies took responsibility for short hauls to and from points inaccessible to motorized ambulances. The Quartermaster Corps provided two animals for each ambulance, and, when not transporting the wounded, they carried fuel and supplies to the dressing stations. These vehicles were slow and presented a vulnerable target when near the front.

In trench warfare, the Medical Department placed two or three motor ambulances, parked at so-called ambulance posts or cabstands, in advance of the dressing station. Safe from the front line, ambulance crews waited on call to transport the wounded. Because of their performance in rough terrain, Fords usually serviced in advance of the dressing station, while the heavier General Motors ambulances were preferred on the roads to the rear. Inevitably, the speed with which ambulance crews evacuated patients depended on the number of casualties, the intensity of artillery fire, the road conditions, the types of available transportation, the status of the patients, and the surgical conditions warranting evacuation.[41]

AMERICAN PREPAREDNESS

Prior to America's entry into the war, army representatives and Red Cross personnel visited universities and medical teaching institutions to recruit physicians, orderlies, and nurses to work in American base-hospital units. Months before the U.S. declaration of war, according to Brigadier General Francis A. Winter, the Red Cross had assembled forty medical units for transfer over to the army. The Red Cross also pulled together large stocks of medical supplies and placed them in warehouses in France prior to the arrival of the U.S. Expeditionary Force. These supplies turned out to be indispensable because of the toll on shipping from submarine warfare. The Medical Department was chronically short of medical supplies and called upon the Red Cross for tents, equipment, and personnel to meet its growing needs. Additionally, the expeditionary force faced an acute shortage of motor ambulances, a shortage assuaged in part by borrowing ambulances from the French and from the Red Cross.[42]

England's request for medical help resulted in the mobilization of six base-hospital units. Colonel J. R. Kean dispatched these units for duty in France with the British Royal Expeditionary Force prior to the arrival of the U.S. Expeditionary Force.[43] The first base hospital to arrive in Europe was organized by George W. Crile, M.D., from personnel from Lakeside Hospital of Western Reserve University in Cleveland, Ohio, and sailed from New York on May 8, 1917. Five more units arrived shortly afterwards from Boston, New York, Philadelphia, St. Louis, and Chicago. All were distributed among the British Royal Expeditionary Force. By armistice, the U.S. Expeditionary Force supported 353,887 beds in France and the United States.[44]

On October 21, 1917, the United States officially entered combat status when it authorized the First U.S. Infantry Division to relieve the French Moroccan Corps in the sector north of Toul between the Saint-Mihiel Salient and the Moselle River. Supporting the division was Evacuation Hospital No. 1, installed in the Sebastopol barracks north of Toul. The German offensive began on March 21, 1918, with a thrust made against the British line north of Montdidier, followed by a wide salient against the French line between the Aisne and Marne rivers. That part of the French line to which the First Division had been assigned performed well against the German army. From that time onward, the conflict raged from the North Sea to Verdun, with the battle at Château-Thierry marking a crucial point in the German drive toward Paris.

Because of the great number of litter bearers killed or wounded by machine-gun and shell fire, medical support units during the battles of Aisne-Marne in June and July 1918 impressed German prisoners into service. Nevertheless, casualties reached such proportions in the early stages of the fighting that medical support units were forced to improvise litters from shirts and jackets with rifles for sidebars. Wounded men remained unattended for days because of the fierceness of the fighting. The lack of drink and food, combined with exhaustion and lowered physical resistance, only worsened their condition. The evacuation circuit clogged as the American medical service was unable to relieve field hospitals of their wounded.[45]

The French army and the U.S. Expeditionary Force worked in close harmony through the war years. American units went into line with French troops, and a subsection of the medical service became known as the *Franco-American section*. Each division of American troops sent to France was supposed to have had two evacuation hospitals; nevertheless, the expeditionary force never realized this level of support and, even after the armistice, no more than 25 percent of the authorized quota was actually in place. Since the Red Cross and other volunteer aid societies had already acquired most of the available buildings suitable for use as hospitals, the United States found it difficult to acquire hospital-type structures except through new construction. Although the French transferred over to the American forces a number of their own hospitals until the Americans were able to construct their own units, most required substantial alterations and additions. After these alterations, however, the hospitals afforded every facility for treating the wounded along modern lines.[46]

The United States built two types of barrack hospitals: the "Type A" unit accommodated one thousand beds, with the potential for a thousand more under emergency conditions; the smaller "Type B" accommodated approximately three hundred beds. These buildings sprang up along the lines of communication—Rimaucourt, Bordeaux, Beaune, Allerey, Mars-la-Tour, Mesves, Limoges, Périgueux, and Nantes. By February 1918, the strength of the U.S. Expeditionary Force approximated a quarter million, with some eleven thousand beds available to serve the sick and wounded and orders to accommodate seventy-three thousand more. By armistice, the American forces were operating 153 base hospitals, 66 camp hospitals, and 12 convalescent camps.[47]

Each division in the U.S. Army operated three ambulance companies, four field hospitals, and two evacuation hospitals. The field hospitals amounted to little more than tents supported with light equipment and their own transportation. Placed as near to the battle as prudent, these hospitals consisted of surgical and shock teams and an operating unit equipped with X-ray machine, steam sterilizer, and other items required for surgical work. Nontransportable cases were treated and retained, while medical personnel transported the remainder to evacuation hospitals or to base hospitals in the rear. As with the British and French medical organizations, the field hospital prepared the wounded for transport to the evacuation hospitals. Of the four hospitals, two were specifically designed for triage to the evacuation hospital, a third was for treatment of gas cases, and a fourth was to treat infectious cases. When fully operational, the evacuation hospitals accommodated a thousand patients and grew considerably larger during times of battle.[48]

The distance between the field ambulance and the evacuation hospital was often more than fifty miles, over nearly impassable terrain cluttered with shell-torn impediments. During the Argonne offensive (September 28 to October 2, 1918), the army ambulance service made the twenty-eight-mile trip from field ambulance to evacuation hospital twenty-four thousand times. In this operation, Evacuation Hospital No. 9 received and evacuated 33,901 cases. Several times each day, the wounded arrived by ambulance car or train and were bathed, fed, dressed, X-rayed, and treated.[49]

General hospitals, such as Twenty-two General Hospital (better known as the "Harvard Unit"), treated both ambulatory and nonambulatory cases. Support staff fed, washed, clothed, classified, cataloged, and distributed wounded to appropriate wards for treatment and care. From there, medical personnel evacuated the patients to convalescent camps and base depots for reclassification or discharge from the army.[50]

In previous wars, hospital ships commissioned to transport sick and wounded were little more than passenger ships altered to accommodate medical, surgical, and infectious cases. During the First World War, most of the belligerents obtained hospital ships in this same fashion, although some built ships especially for the purpose. When the United States declared war, it had only one navy hospital ship in commission and two under construction. The United States Surgeon General's Office estimated that 7 percent of the total American forces in France would return each year as sick and wounded. Of that percentage, half would be bed cases. Because of these numbers, the United States employed troop-transport ships to return many of the sick and wounded.[51]

SANITARY TRAINS

For the whole of Europe, whose population between 1871 and 1914 had grown from 293 to 490 million and whose economic expansion had shown similarly dramatic increases, the railway offered the most efficient and effective solution to transportation needs in both peace and war. Although railroads would prove difficult to use in areas close to the front, rail lines conclusively and repeatedly demonstrated their usefulness. While the internal-combustion engine introduced motorized vehicles into the war, thereby providing greater mobility and tactical control, the railroad, animal-drawn vehicles, and the legs of men remained the predominant forms of transportation during the war.[52]

Ambulance trains were of three types: *permanent*, *ordinary*, and *improvised*. The permanent ambulance trains were built and equipped to carry the most serious cases. These trains consisted of ambulance coaches, fitted with tiers of cots; coaches for sitting patients; and cars for dispensary, kitchen, operating theater, support personnel, and supplies. Temporary hospital trains consisted of ordinary coaches and rolling stock, which had been fitted with special apparatus, such as the Zavodovsky system (cables stretched across the coach from which stretchers were hung) and the Brechot-Deprez-Ameline system (an iron framework mounted on springs that carried three stretchers), to accommodate the wounded. The Royal Army Medical Corps installed Brechot-Deprez-Ameline sets in empty railway cars to carry twelve recumbent cases. Improvised hospital trains transported supplies and troops to the front and evacuated wounded during heavy engagements as, for example, the Decauville light-railway system, which carried ammunition from the railhead to the guns and returned with wounded from advanced dressing stations.[53]

During the battle of the Marne in the early months of the war, soldiers spoke of yet another train that, by any definition, was hardly sanitary. Freight cars strewn with straw and third-class carriages with stretchers lashed to the seats served as makeshift transport. Worse still, cars used to transport horses to the front carried thousands of wounded from the battle area. Because there was no opportunity to clean and disinfect these cars, many of the wounded developed tetanus and gas gangrene afterwards.[54]

Initially, sanitary trains lacked connecting sections, restricting surgeons to a single car; this meant that the wounded traveled without medical aid unless the train made intermittent stops to permit emergency care. Although stops allowed surgeons and attendants to provide this care, the delays usually offset the benefits. The system had worked in the vast distances of the South African war, but the circumstances in France were hardly comparable. Delays simply increased the incidence of sepsis and further exhausted the wounded. Eventually, communicating doorways, built at each end of the car, provided needed access from one end of the train to the other, allowing surgeons and medical attendants to tend to the wounded without stopping.[55]

The British ambulance train service began August 17, 1914, with a gift from the French of one hundred merchandise wagons, a few passenger coaches, and some luggage vans. Medical personnel divided the donated cars into three separate trains (numbered 1, 2, and 3), disinfected them, outfitted them with the Brechot-Deprez-Ameline apparatus, added kitchens, staffed them with medical support personnel, and moved them to the front. Next, they provisioned a fourth train out of third-class passenger carriages after having removed the seats. Another train, donated by the French government and christened the *Franco-British*, began operating in early September. There being no motor ambulances in France at this time, the wounded were moved to the trains in animal carts or motor supply wagons belonging to the Royal Army Service Corps.[56]

Medical personnel introduced additional trains into service as soon as carriages, vans, and other moving stock became available. By September 20, 1914, seven ambulance trains, each able to accommodate approximately two hundred cases, were running between the front and the base hospitals or ports (plates 51, 52). By October 30, two additional trains came into service, while the Red Cross and the St. John of Jerusalem Society were fitting yet another ambulance train at Sotteville-lès-Rouen. These trains were supported by two medical officers, three nursing sisters, and forty-five noncommissioned officers and men, and they carried upwards of eight hundred casualties.[57]

After April 1915, the British began constructing ambulance trains in their own yards and factories. Nevertheless, of the first twelve British trains placed in service, eleven were made from railway carriages donated by the French government. Between August 1914 and April 1915, sixty-seven thousand of England's wounded traveled to evacuation ports in France by way of these twelve ambulance trains.[58]

At English ports, the pressures created by the large numbers of sick and wounded arriving from France proved nearly overwhelming, forcing medical personnel to seek various extemporized means of converting vehicles to carry stretcher cases. After attempting several arrangements, including the classic Zavodovsky system, they successfully tested an economical folding trestle that would hold two stretchers between each pair of trestles. Built entirely of wood, the trestles facilitated easy packing for transport and improvised quickly in various carriages. In all, some twenty-eight army and four naval trains (consisting of nine to sixteen cars) operated in England and Scotland, moving wounded from ports to hospitals throughout Great Britain.[59]

Initially, the American army considered adapting ordinary supply cars for hospital trains, fitting them with supporting tiers similar to those used during the Civil War and the Franco-Prussian War. The supporting tiers consisted of metal posts connected to both roof and floor that medical personnel could build quickly. In practice, however, the delays incurred in constructing the tiers resulted in unnecessary suffering for the sick and wounded. Moreover, sanitary personnel required additional time to clean the cars and to collect food and other supplies for the trip. Only in emergencies, usually after a major engagement, did the sanitary corps utilize ordinary coaches or rolling stock.[60] The U.S. Expeditionary Force profited from the French and British experience by authorizing the construction of standard hospital trains to meet its needs. The United States ordered forty-eight such hospital trains built in England, although most arrived too late to be used in the war. In their place, the Americans depended upon borrowed French trains, many of which were simply boxcars.[61]

By 1918, the Americans had seventeen complete hospital trains (272 coaches) in service. Each train, composed of sixteen coaches, contained one infectious-case car (eighteen beds), one staff car, one kitchen and sitting sick-officers' car, eight ordinary lying ward cars (288 beds), one pharmacy car, one infectious sitting car, one kitchen and mess car, one personnel car, and one train-crew and storage car. On average, the American hospital trains supported four hundred beds each. Electrically lighted and steam heated, they provided ample accommodations for the wounded and support personnel in the evacuation process. The Red Cross on a white background was prominently displayed on each side of every coach; some trains also had the Red Cross painted on the roof for identification by aircraft.[62]

On their way to special hospitals across the United States, 65,289 sick and wounded soldiers passed through New York City. From the debarkation hospitals, which acted as clearinghouses for the wounded, sanitary corpsmen sorted out the patients and distributed them to interior hospitals. Hospital trains regularly left Grand Central Station in New York for Fort Kearney, San Diego, Chicago, and other parts of the country. The typical hospital train consisted of twenty-four special hospital-unit cars; on occasion, however, sanitary personnel simply attached hospital cars to regular trains for the journey.[63]

Although military and sanitary personnel expressed initial skepticism toward the practicality, reliability, and durability of motorized transport (other than trains) in war, the experiences of the First World War proved emphatically that motorized armies had become a vital part of warfare.

Between the horse-drawn wagon, which remained the mainstay of the embattled armies on all fronts, and the highly publicized introduction of the airplane and dirigible, the steady increase in the production and deployment of motorized transport presaged a whole new stage in military planning and operations. Gasoline-powered vehicles proved as valuable for evacuating wounded men as they were for the tactical movement of men, supplies, and reinforcements to and from the front. Medical planners now had their choice of supporting wounded soldiers close to the firing line or in safe areas more distant from the guns—a choice that became increasingly important as medical corpsmen and evacuees came under air attack and long-range artillery. The paradigm of the horse-drawn wagon had shifted; modern warfare and the technology for swift and decisive evacuation of the wounded had finally come of age.

7

Lessons Learned

Except for the ebullient Americans, who touted their short, intense, aggressive efforts as decisive for the Allies, victory came as a muted triumph for the governments and peoples who had joined the patriotic cause of August 1914. For these belligerents, the war became a labyrinth of manufactured horror and indecisiveness. Few nations remained untouched by the slaughter, and the stillness that hung over Europe in its aftermath left little room for Wilsonian idealism; instead, nations sought security from each other's weaknesses. Although few medical planners believed that nations would deliberately choose to fight another siege war, they found themselves in a quandary as they looked at the alternatives. Because the Great War had provided their single most significant experience, planners found themselves drawn to its statistics as they calculated distances between evacuation points, analyzed the profile of casualties and the average period for their hospitalization, counted the numbers of temporary and permanent beds in the zone of the interior, noted the location and effectiveness of medical railheads, and speculated on the potential role of the air ambulance. Only slowly did planners redefine their evacuation strategies in the context of maturing tactics and technology.

Medical personnel had assumed at the beginning of the First World War that military operations would involve rapid movement, that the number of serious casualties would be fewer than in previous wars, and that belligerents would honor the Geneva Convention in protecting the wounded. Each of these assumptions proved dreadfully wrong. In prior wars, the ratio of those killed to wounded averaged 1:4, a ratio very much determined by the mode of attack. Trench warfare, with its heavy emphasis on shells and other explosive missiles, increased the ratio of killed to wounded—a change that had already been witnessed in the Turko-Balkan War of 1912–13, where the ratio of killed to wounded was 1:2.5. While the ratio remained about 1:4.2 for the American fighting troops in the Great War, trench fighting on the western front brought the ratio to 1:3 for the French, 1:2.9 for the British, and 1:2.8 for the Germans. Also, in contrast to previous wars, the number of instantaneous deaths increased, owing to high explosives and the resulting massive hemorrhages in the central nervous system and lungs. Then, too, the nature of casualties changed dramatically from prewar estimates. Despite horrendous bacteriological problems, battle casualties on the western front up to the armistice exceeded the number of deaths from communicable diseases. Tetanus, typhoid fever, and dysentery, which had been the scourge of armies since earliest times, were reduced significantly through rigid sanitation and vaccinations. Not until 1917–19, when the Spanish influenza swept across Europe and the United States, did the mortality figures from disease become more devastating. The eastern front, however, continued to reflect casualty figures of earlier conflicts; there, armies faced high incidences of contagious diseases throughout the conflict, especially exanthematous typhus and cholera.[1]

Another assumption that proved erroneous for the warring nations was that wounds from steel-jacketed bullets would be clean, requiring a simple first dressing to seal the wound. Medical planners based their assumption on field experiences in the Boer War, where 90 percent of the wounds came from bullet penetrations and where the combatants moved over largely uncultivated lands. In contrast, soldiers in the Great War fought in the plowed soil of the Champagne where 85 percent of the wounds resulted from high-explosive shells or grenades and where even minor wounds became infected. Shell fragments tore small holes in the skin and connective tissues but literally exploded muscle fiber, tearing vessels, killing cells by molecular shock, and filling the wound area with bloody fluid in which dead and dying cells, dirt, and bits of clothing mingled to create an ideal environment for infection; every soldier was a bacillus carrier. Fecal organisms, especially sporebearing anaerobic microbes responsible for gas gangrene and tetanus, established themselves in the wound.

Not surprisingly, wounded who were left unattended for days on the battlefield or whose transport was interrupted for extended periods by artillery barrages faced life-threatening infections, which passed into nonsporing bacteria (i.e., streptococci and *Proteus*) and pyogenic cocci. The mortality rate from tetanus soared to over 70 percent for soldiers who did not receive antitoxin. No longer could surgeons regard any wound as clean, as they found themselves actively preventing and controlling infection—through antiseptic pastes, salt packs, and wound irrigation, debridement or wound excision, and primary suture.[2]

Both German and Allied armies experienced a disproportionately high number of gunshot fractures among their battle-wounded. Fractures acounted for nearly 8 percent of the total number of wounds, roughly 15 percent of which required surgical intervention because of extensive bone damage. With high-velocity bullets came wounds that appeared to have been caused by an "explosion" within the tissue. Although external signs of injury were slight, with small entrance and exit holes, the tissues pulped within and about the bullet path, and bones shattered without even suffering a direct hit. Theories that the "wind" or "shock wave" produced the special cavitation or explosive effect of the wound proved false on closer examination. The same was true for theories based on the rotary motion of the rifled muzzle, the flattening of the bullet, and the heating effect as the bullet passed through tissue. Instead, scientists focused on the "accelerated-particle" theory, which regarded "the energy of the bullet as being transferred to the soft tissue in front and to each side, thus imparting momentum to these tissue particles, so that they rapidly move away from the bullet path, thus acting as 'secondary missiles.'"[3] Damage was caused not just by the bullet but also by the fluids moving away from the bullet's path. L. B. Wilson compared this "blasting" out of tissues to the effect that a stream of water from a fire hose has upon soft material.[4]

Of course, the rifle bullet, however destructive, played a secondary role to artillery projectiles, bombs, and grenade fragments. Although lacking velocity and penetrating power, these latter weapons almost invariably carried fragments of clothing and other foreign materials into the wound, rendering it septic. The rifle bullet did not do nearly as much wounding in the Great War as it had in previous wars, and given the trench-style tactics in France and Flanders, the septic wound assumed an importance not seen in earlier experiences in Manchuria in the Russo-Japanese War, in Egypt and Palestine, and in the South African war. In both the Spanish-American and South African wars, shell and shrapnel wounds accounted for between 5 percent and 10 percent of the total gunshot wounds. In the Russo-Japanese War, shell wounds were 14 percent, while in the Turko-Balkan War of 1912–13, shell and shrapnel wounds averaged about one-third of the total wounded. Thus, remarked M. W. Ireland, "the ratio of gunshot wounds formerly obtaining, in which the wounds caused by rifle missiles were typical, became reversed [in World War I] and so found surgeons in a state of unpreparedness."[5]

The resulting necrosis from shrapnel became an ideal medium for pathogenic bacteria and, under such conditions, wound contamination became the rule rather than the exception. Even strong antiseptics provided little benefit. Not until Alexis Carrel, René Lemaître, and H. M. W. Gray reintroduced the principle of excision (debridement) of the devitalized necrotic portions of the wounds did surgeons reduce the danger of infection. Following extensive debate at the Interallied Surgical Conference in Paris in 1917, surgeons agreed to reassess the high mortality of primary wound closure and institute open-wound treatment and secondary closure of contaminated wounds. By the end of the war, wound excision followed by delayed wound closure had become established practices of front-line surgery.[6]

The combatants in the Great War learned that most battle wounds became infected regardless of correct application of the first field dressing. This reality reinforced the need to treat all wounds within twelve to thirty-six hours and to examine all casualties according to modern surgical practice prior to their removal to the base hospital. Along with recognition that the wounded required the most rapid means of transport, these two principles formed the basis of medical planning in the 1920s. This meant making every effort to avoid delays at the *postes de secours* or other areas for lack of appropriate transportation.[7]

The introduction late in the war of gas shells, small-caliber field guns carried by the infantry, and a new type of light machine gun enabled troops to advance rapidly over the battlefield without waiting for field or heavy artillery. This, too, forced unavoidable changes in the positioning of hospitals and other sanitary support units behind the lines. Unless defenders could respond quickly with reinforcements to the front trenches, and unless backed by sufficient fire power, sanitary support had to fall back until the lines stabilized. Rapid advances threatened field ambulances with loss or capture, forcing medical units to transport the wounded thirty to fifty miles by train or motor ambulance before giving them any surgical dressing other than first aid. This delay meant that fatalities from shock, hemorrhage, peritonitis, and gas gangrene increased to inexcusable proportions.

The French, who preferred large hospital centers, found their system both economical and responsive as long as the battlefield shifted no more than one to five miles on either side. However, the change in March 1918 to a war of movement brought an abrupt end to this system, as the larger sanitary units were unable to react quickly to the destabilization of the front. In contrast, smaller units found it easier to fall back to more secure locations on short notice. The offensives of 1918 taught both the French and the British that large evacuation hospitals or hospital centers situated eight to fifteen miles from the front would "almost inevitably either be captured, forced to evacuate very hurriedly on account of shelling or aerial bombing, or rendered useless because of the impossibility of headquarters forseeing, from hour to hour or even from day to day, just where the battle line would become stabilized."[8] Although several British C.C.S.s fell into German hands, they remained operational until the very last moment of evacuation. This was not true for the French, whose hospital centers in the same sector spent fifteen days packing and unpacking their equipment, following orders and countermanded orders to retreat. At the height of the battle, these hospitals were utterly useless, unable to provide needed support to the wounded.

Another lesson learned from this experience was that large hospital units required locations near railheads. Unfortunately, these units came increasingly under heavy shelling and aerial bombardment because of their proximity to munitions and other military stores requiring the same rail connections.[9]

The change from a stationary war to a war of movement, according to Major George de Tarnowsky, necessitated large numbers of "small rapidly mobile surgical units, capable of operating upon relatively large numbers of cases and supplied with constant, rapid means of transportation." The small mobile units could move on short notice, had better control over personnel and wounded, and could be located in areas safe from discovery by the enemy. Thus, the mobile unit became an advanced operating room, minimizing complications due to potential delay in treatment. In de Tarnowsky's proposed system, each evacuation hospital would maintain three to five mobile units of eighty to one hundred beds and work in close cooperation with motor ambulances. De Tarnowsky suggested that mobile medical teams could treat severe hemorrhage; edema of the glottis; intra-abdominal lesions; intracranial lesions; intrathoracic wounds with shell fragment in situ; wound shock; fractures by immobilizing them; and penetrating or perforating shell wounds of the arm, forearm, buttocks, thigh, and calf. Evacuations from the mobile units occurred once or twice every twenty-four hours.[10]

De Tarnowsky's recommendations notwithstanding, the U.S. Expeditionary Force chose to retain its structure of three ambulance companies, four mobile field hospitals, and two evacuation hospitals for each division. According to Chief Surgeon A. N. Stark, First Army, the difficulties of administration and supply and the uneconomical use of medical support personnel would more than offset the advantages of several additional mobile units. And unless provided with special transportation, Stark predicted that they would not necessarily retain their mobility.[11]

Physicians concluded from their wartime experiences that field hospitals should be prepared to operate on the seriously wounded, particularly those with chest and abdominal wounds, as well as provide transfusions, stabilize shock victims, and perform amputations. Accordingly, medical teams required the most modern surgical equipment in the field hospitals and insisted that operating teams be ready to provide immediate support.[12]

Because of their size and organization, medical detachments—which at times were forced to evacuate up to half of the personnel of a regiment— proved to be ineffective during the war. This meant that larger medical detachments, not combat troops, would be needed to provide aid and carry litters. The war also demonstrated the acute shortage of ambulances and other evacuation support between division and evacuation hospitals. Following the war, new tables of organization included a greater number of personnel detached to medical units, the abolition of sanitary trains, an improvement in communications between and among aid stations by field telephones, and the addition of the air ambulance.[13]

Above all else, medical personnel who had experienced the horrendous numbers of battle-wounded arriving from the front recognized the importance of triage as the most effective methodological selection system for classifying the sick and wounded. This selection process, designed to function under conditions of high pressure during and after periods of battle, required trained teams of doctors and support personnel who were both willing to make, and capable of making, quick and correct decisions and to follow up those decisions with an orderly, competent, and energetic response. Its value lay in arranging cases for treatment and maintaining a careful balance between the urgency of hospitalization and the need for orderly evacuation. Under the pressure of such emergencies, indecision meant the difference between lifesaving intervention for those patients for whom intervention had a reasoned chance of success and an undisciplined and unmethodological approach, which threatened the life and safety of patients and wasted valuable human resource efforts. Triage became an internationally recognized battlefield support system that, while leading to standardization, left each nation with enough latitude to adjust its details to the traditions of its unique military and medical organization.[14]

A great deal of planning in the mid 1920s focused on intercommunication between the medical formations and the front lines, as well as on better coordination within and among medical units. Discussions dealt with telephone systems, visual signals, radios, runners, mounted dispatch riders, cyclists, and other methods of improving communication in a war of movement. Military planners especially encouraged medical officers to become involved in war operations, to carry out exercises of medical tactics on maps as well as on the ground, and to react more responsively to decision making. Advocated in 1917 by Edward L. Munson, in *The Principles of Sanitary Tactics*, this plan did not achieve full endorsement until after the war. Nonetheless, Munson's advice remained relevant.

> Maneuvers in the field bring into play a factor which must of necessity be disregarded in the theoretical study of tactics, both general and sanitary, and which falls peculiarly within the purview and study of duty of the medical officer. This relates to the physical ability of troops to perform the various tasks to which they are set in the solution of problems and execution of tactical and sanitary plans. This factor is largely dependent upon the hygienic care of troops, which is the first duty with which the Medical Department is charged in peace and war. It is an intangible quality which is readily apparent to the trained observer, though not to be expressed on paper any more than can the mental state which may stimulate to victory on the one hand or result in disorganization, defeat and rout on the other. It is true that well-conceived plans, worked out by leaders, are necessary to success, whether tactical or sanitary—but the final and controlling factor is, after all, the quality of ability to execute military purpose possessed by the men behind the guns.[15]

Major General John F. Morrison's and Lieutenant Edward L. Munson's *Study in Troop Leading and Management of Sanitary Service in War* (1918) represented an effort by the Army School of the Line to simulate conditions of battle and the close coordination required between the leading of troops and the management of a sanitary service. Planned originally as a study in battle orders, the manual provided a more precise delineation of the functions and purposes of the Medical Department and the duties expected of medical officers in an active campaign. Using Fort

Leavenworth and its vicinity as the reference point for the tactical and sanitary positions cited in the text, the authors provided graphic examples of the organizing principles that constituted a successful military and medical operation. Beginning with an overview of the general prebattle situation, the authors proceeded to lead the student officer through the tactical situation and preliminary measures taken by the Medical Department; through the daylight battles and management of sanitary personnel and equipment during this period; through the cessation of battle and partial sanitation of the battlefield by relief agencies; and, finally, through the service of security, information, and shelter of the army, accompanied by the completion of the battlefield's sanitation and the evacuation of the wounded.[16]

During the 1920s, planning and sanitary personnel focused primarily on wars of movement, recognizing that the stationary nature of the Great War did not preclude a more active disposition of armies. In addition, they concerned themselves with the need for protecting medical units from both machine-gun and field-artillery fire, protecting units and wounded from enemy movement, carefully gauging the distances between front lines and aid stations, and ensuring that all combatants respected the Geneva Convention.[17]

Although the war forced the military in nearly every country to think almost exclusively of motorized ambulances and railroads in the evacuation of their sick and wounded, their experiences did not remove entirely the need for animal-drawn ambulances or, for that matter, dependence on native transportation. In the Philippine Islands during the 1920s, the United States Army Medical Corps chose to rely on the carreta or drag, the sled, the carabao cart, the carretela, and the calesa or carromata. The drag, or carreta, resembled the travois used earlier by the American Indian and by United States Army personnel attached to the western service. Consisting of two long poles fastened together by several wooden slats and attached to the yoke of an animal, the carreta provided transportation over terrain considered impassable for wheeled vehicles. The sled, constructed of bamboo, differed little from that used on American farms for hauling supplies in muddy areas. The carabao cart, the carretela, and the calesa were two-wheeled carts drawn by an ox or by a native pony and served multiple duties in the islands. The calesa accommodated sitting cases, while the carretela supported recumbent patients. Aside from these types of transport, medical corpsmen also employed the two-horse litter typical of the earlier western service.[18]

The Great War witnessed significant wartime contributions in neurology, ophthalmology, military hygiene, pathology, and roentgenology.

Other areas that benefited from the war experience included the physi-
ological aspects of aviation, improved control of wound tetanus, pathology and treatment of gas poisoning, introduction of deep antisepsis,
rehabilitation of the crippled and blind, and work with the shell-shocked.
The constant bombardment of the trenches had resulted in unusually
high rates of shell shock. Although not visibly injured by the bombs and
artillery, soldiers suffered blindness; loss of memory, taste, and smell;
impaired hearing; and other physical symptoms. As for "wound shock,"
the war resulted in a full review of shock theories, as well as suggestions
for treatment, including checking for hemorrhage, administering hot
drinks (except for those with abdominal wounds), raising the legs to
improve circulation, injecting stimulants, such as strychnine and vaso-
constrictive drugs (pituitrin and adrenalin), experimenting with forced
absorption of fluids, injecting salt and gum-salt solutions, and undertaking blood transfusions. During the latter part of the war, medical officers
received instruction on the nature of shock, the theories concerning its
onset, its clinical manifestations, the conditions and principles of its
treatment, and the important work of shock teams and resuscitation
officers in the shock ward.[19]

Post–World War I surgical congresses focused on hemostasis, wound
infection, plastic surgery of the face and jaw, dental reconstruction,
protection from gas edema, open-wound treatment, antisepsis of deep
tissues using quinine derivatives, the manufacture of artificial limbs, and
gunshot wounds to the spinal cord. Doctors also shared information on
nerve suture, improved vascular surgery, new techniques with splints and
bandages, surgical measures in gunshot wounds of the skull and abdomen, the extraction of foreign bodies from the eye, and serotherapy in
internal medicine.

Etiological findings and diagnoses represented some of the brightest
accomplishments of the war: surgeons gained new insight into the
investigation of gunshot wounds to the abdomen; the use of stereoscopic
photographs to locate foreign bodies; the rise in microscopic and cultural
investigations in the bacteriological diagnoses of the dysenteries; and the
importance of early diagnosis of syphilis. Sanitary personnel demonstrated the successful, widespread use of preventative inoculations against
typhoid, cholera, and paratyphoid; the preventative inoculation of tetanus serum immediately after the infliction of a wound; and the recognition of latent infection in tetanus and in gas gangrene. Also from their
wartime experiences, surgeons and sanitary personnel developed a better
understanding of shock and the predisposing causes of trench foot. In
addition, they learned more regarding the early intervention of surgery

and transfusion to halt hemorrhage, the importance of rapid transportation of the wounded, the expectation of at least 25-percent casualties in any attack, the need for a competent field hospital capable of full medical service and excellent communication from the front lines to more distant evacuation hospitals.[20]

THE AIR AMBULANCE

The first reference in literature to the air ambulance was Jules Verne's *Robur le Conquérant* (1866), which describes the rescue of shipwrecked men by the airship *Albatros*. According to Harry George Armstrong, in *Principles and Practice of Aviation Medicine* (1952), doctors used observation balloons to evacuate 160 sick during the siege of Paris in 1870. From 1890 to 1910, Chief of the Dutch Medical Service M. de Mooy (known as "the Jules Verne of air-ambulance service") advocated a method of transporting the sick and wounded using stretchers suspended from balloons. French Senator Emile Raymond, a medical doctor and aviator who died during an air reconnaissance flight in the early days of World War I, and Mille. Marvingt, a colleague of de Mooy, proposed aerial ambulance support for the military as early as 1912. During the Poitou maneuvers in September of that year, Raymond flew over the battlefield in a Bleriot and simulated the identification of casualties for stretcher parties. In October 1913, French medical officer M. Gautier commented that "we shall revolutionize war surgery if the aeroplane can be adapted as a means of transport for the wounded." A similar reference occurred at the *Société de Medécin Militaire* in 1913, when M. Uzac and Charles Julliot of the French *Service de Santé* urged the extension of the Geneva Convention to air-ambulance support.[21]

Independent of these French initiatives, Captain George H. R. Gosman of the U.S. Army Medical Corps and Lieutenant Albert L. Rhoades of the Coast Artillery Corps collaborated in 1909 at Pensacola, Florida, to design and build a plane for aeromedical evacuation. Their design required the pilot to be a doctor and to sit next to the patient while flying the plane. During its maiden flight, however, the plane encountered mechanical problems and crashed. Lacking funds to continue and viewed by the War Department as peripheral to the needs of the military, Gosman and Rhoades halted their experiments. Three years later, Secretary of War Henry L. Stimson reiterated the position of the War Department when he opposed the use of airplanes to transport military patients. Despite his disapproval, Colonel A. W. Williams recommended that airplanes be used to transport wounded soldiers from the battlefield to general hospitals. This suggestion, which Williams made to the Committee on Transportation of the Association of Military Surgeons in Baltimore in November 1912, would later prove relevant to military discussions in the 1920s.[22]

During the Serbian army's retreat from the Albanian mountains in November 1915, a Captain Dangelzer and a Lieutenant Paulhan of the French squadron successfully evacuated wounded men from Mitrovica to Prizren and then to Vallona by air. Not until 1917 did French Surgeon A. Chassaing, working with Justin Godart, improvise space in the fuselage of the Dorant AR II military plane to evacuate stretcher cases from the Soissons sector. Soon afterwards, Chassaing had six airplanes at his disposal, and in April 1918, two of these planes assisted in the evacuation from Flanders. These two examples appear to be the only recorded instances of aerial ambulance evacuation in the war, the British having decided that such evacuation was unnecessary. Nevertheless, Chassaing proved the practicality of aeromedical evacuation and, following the war, was assigned to Morocco, where the French government gave him sixty Bréguet 14-2-A–type airplanes for conversion to ambulance duty. By 1920, he had twenty planes available for duty in Morocco and another sixteen in the Levant. By 1921, all sixty airplanes were in regular use. With the gun turret removed and a side door constructed in the fuselage to admit two stretchers, the Bréguet XIV-T machine adapted easily to medical evacuation. Known as the "father of ambulance aeroplanes," Chassaing saw his ideas spread worldwide by the end of the 1920s.[23]

The French continued to expand upon the idea of the aerial ambulance during brief campaigns in Morocco and Syria between 1921 and 1925. There, the French established the Medical Air Transport Service under a Colonel Cheutin. There, too, the French introduced the *aérochir*, a medical support system that enabled surgeons and personnel to proceed by plane to where the wounded lay. The *aérochir* did not prove effective: it was more important to move the wounded to the safety of hospital facilities than to have medical personnel move to the field, leaving behind valuable medical equipment. For transporting the wounded, the French utilized the large Bréguet-Limousine aircraft, capable of carrying eight to ten cases, and the smaller Hanriot biplane, which fitted two stretcher cases through a lateral porthole in the fuselage. Pilots especially appreciated the Hanriot because of its ability to land and take off on short runways and because of its durability. It performed well in evacuating the wounded to dressing stations twenty miles behind the line, where the Bréguet then carried them to base hospitals. By 1929, the Moroccan Air Medical Service consisted of seventeen Hanriots and twenty-six Bréguet-type planes.[24]

In 1923, the French Ministry of War, in collaboration with the French Air Service and the Army Medical Corps, evacuated seven hundred wounded men by air ambulances to hospitals in Meknès, Fès, and Casablanca at distances ranging from 50 to 350 miles. By 1925, the French service had transported more than three thousand sick and wounded soldiers by air in Morocco and Syria. These experiences demonstrated conclusively to the French the value of the aerial ambulance, particularly that it was neither more dangerous nor more costly than ground transportation. More importantly, it proved timesaving, reduced mortality, and improved troop morale. The aerial ambulance not only shortened the time taken to transport wounded soldiers from the front to hospitals but also permitted sanitary personnel to evacuate the wounded from remote regions controlled by dissident tribes. At Wargla (Ouargla), in the countryside of southern Algeria, the French medical corps borrowed airplanes belonging to the bombing squadron to transport surgeons to dressing stations and to evacuate the wounded to hospitals hundreds of miles away.[25]

Although the first British aeromedical evacuation occurred at Bir-el-Hassana in the Sinai Desert in February 1917, there was a reluctance to repeat this initial success.[26] In January 1920, Captain J. C. Burnjs of the R.A.M.C. witnessed a further demonstration of aeromedical evacuation when a British officer, with a bullet wound to the liver, was transported in an R.E.8 two-seater from the village of Abukemal to Baghdad 260 miles away.[27] The British eventually overcame their reluctance to test the air ambulance during their occupation of the Iraq Protectorate in 1923, when they experimented with the Vickers-Vernon in trial flights from Kirkuk to Baghdad, a distance of 185 miles. They also airlifted 198 cases of acute dysentery out of the Kurdistan Mountains; using Vickers-Vernon troop carriers, pilots made 95 flights over a period of 128 hours to evacuate patients to hospitals in Baghdad. Soon afterwards, the British routinely transported cases by air—the 625 miles from Baghdad to Egypt—a journey that took three to four weeks by land. They also tested a navy stretcher that, known affectionately as the "mummy case," strapped to the fuselage of a Bristol fighter, 9A, or Vickers-Vimy. The British later developed the Avro-Andover, which carried two recumbent and two sitting patients, and the Vermont-Victoria, which carried twenty-four sitting or fourteen recumbent patients. By 1929, the Vermont-Victoria had become the standard British air ambulance.[28]

Those strategists who looked to future wars saw an extended use of airplanes in the medical services. Although not considered useful near the front lines, particularly in a siege war, their applicability in a war of movement was clearly recognized. According to Air Commodore David Munro in 1923, the air ambulance could evacuate men suffering severe head and abdominal injuries. The British even considered establishing an air-ambulance convoy similar to the motor-ambulance convoy. Despite these visionary efforts, as late as 1931 England still had no organized medical transport service. Instead, it settled for a collection of voluntary flying personnel, organized under the auspices of the British Red Cross Society and sanctioned by the Air Ministry.[29]

At the International Conference of the Red Cross in 1923, delegates debated whether the aerial ambulance could be effective in war and, if so, what forms of protection the belligerent powers should extend to it. The results became the basis for a commission that submitted its findings to the International Conference of the Red Cross in Geneva in 1925. The commission prepared a supplement to the Geneva Convention of 1906 recognizing the protection of medical units whose equipment was used exclusively for the transport of the sick and wounded or for the transport of its own personnel and medical stores. The statement prohibited medical aircraft from having signaling devices, weapons, or photographic capability. Moreover, unless agreed upon by the belligerent powers, the convention statement prohibited air ambulances from flying over, or even approaching, the battle line. To ensure the safety of air-ambulance transport, the statement recommended that air corps identify the name and number of each plane used to transport sick and wounded men. While the machines were not subject to capture, they were open to inspection. Finally, the statement directed all nations using air ambulances to paint their aircraft white and place the Red Cross insignia above and below the wings and on both sides of the fuselage.[30]

American Air-Ambulance Service

In the November 1918 issue of *Annals of Surgery*, Norvelle Wallace Sharpe, M.D., a captain in the U.S. Medical Corps, suggested the design of an "ambulance airship" constructed from a Curtiss JN4D biplane. He envisaged an airship that, with distinctive Red Cross markings on the wings and sides, would operate in the "zone of the advance" to recover downed pilots. He suggested that air rescue involve two planes: one to serve as the ambulance airship, stocked with appropriate first-aid dressings and tools (axe, bolt cutter, and saw) to remove the pilot from the crash, and the other to assist in the search. To ensure quick response to downed pilots, Sharpe recommended that the U.S. Army Air Corps develop its own ambulance service rather than rely upon other service organizations.[31]

Sharpe's suggestion was not too different from that of Captain William C. Ocker, officer in charge of flight training at Gerstner Field in Louisiana, and Major Wilson E. Driver, who proposed that an "aeroambulance" with a physician on board be sent to aid injured pilots. After providing first aid, the pilot would transport the injured flyer to Gerstner Hospital for treatment. This model was subsequently put into service at the Taylor, Post, Mather, Rich, and Carruthers fields.[32] In 1919, Major S. M. Strong of the United States Army Medical Corps noted the value of transporting patients by aircraft and designed an aeroambulance for use at Eberts Field in Arkansas. The ambulance consisted of a remodeled Curtiss biplane, which accommodated a single litter in place of the rear cockpit (plates 53, 54).[33]

Following the war, the U.S. Army Air Corps took a particular interest in the aerial transportation of the sick and wounded and, under the guidance of its chief surgeon, Colonel Albert E. Truby, studied the suitability of existing planes for ambulance work. As a consequence of that study, the service's engineering division modified the DeHaviland DH-4A to accommodate a pilot, a medical officer, and two patients. The U.S. Army Air Corps used this modified air ambulance for crash-rescue service in the Southwest during the 1920s and supplemented it with the Curtiss Eagle for longer-range air evacuation.[34]

By the mid to late 1920s, United States military planners concluded that the air ambulance should become "a means of normal evacuation in modern wars." L. H. Bauer, M.D., medical director of aeronautics in the United States Department of Commerce, and his Europpean counterparts recognized that the air ambulance would force a reconsideration of sanitary-support organization and services. This reconsideration included the need to locate aircraft within close proximity of battles, so that the machines could fly to the front lines; the need to build hospitals close to airfields; the applicability of the Geneva Convention to sanitary aircraft; the conversion of commercial airplanes into evacuation ambulances; the desirability of amphibian planes for ambulance support; the types of wounds that would benefit from air transportation; and the neutralization of ambulance aircraft in time of war.[35]

On July 1, 1925, the army created the Medical Section of the Office of the Chief of the Army Air Corps to develop an air-ambulance service for the army. Although the earliest air ambulances consisted of refitted military planes, in January 1926, the army provided specially built planes for Kelly Field in Texas, France Field in Panama, and March Field in California. Shortly afterward, the United States made its first military use of the air ambulance by providing medical supplies and then evacuating eighteen sick and wounded marines from jungle garrisons in Nicaragua, 150 miles from medical support units.

Within a few short years, the army had equipped most of its Air Corps stations with air ambulances, which transported patients tens of thousands of miles each year. One popular air ambulance was the Fokker, stationed at Wright Field in Ohio in 1931 and later at Randolph Field. The Fokker Corporation designed its air ambulance for speeds of 133 miles per hour and equipped it with extralarge balloon tires, shock absorbers, and space for transporting three litter patients and a flight surgeon. The plane also contained surgical supplies, lavatory, and thermos bottles and was heated to minimize the trauma of shock.[36] By the 1930s, American medical strategists were designing air ambulances powered by more than one engine, with heated cabin, cruising speed of one hundred miles per hour, fuel capacity for six hours, room for six litters or ten sitting cases, and short-runway capability. Military planners considered the air ambulance's greatest usefulness in connecting the larger military hospitals, such as Walter Reed, Letterman, and Beaumont, by means of these "ships of mercy."[37]

On the basis of the Meuse-Argonne battle statistics, strategists in the 1930s predicted a 6-percent casualty rate per battle day for a division of 21,500 men; 3 percent for a corps of 90,100; and 1.5 percent for an army of 325,000. Of these numbers, they also estimated that one in six would be killed, leaving as wounded 1,075, or 5 percent of a division; 2,250, or 2.5 percent of a corps; and 4,060, or 1.25 percent of an army, all requiring some level of medical attention. Of those numbers, the categories of wounded fell into 25 percent, or 270, slightly wounded, who would require transportation to evacuation hospitals using motorized ground ambulances, and 75 percent, or 805, more seriously wounded, who would need evacuation to general hospitals by air ambulances. Computing the distance from the forward landing field to the field adjacent to a general hospital as approximately seventy-five miles, with each ambulance carrying an average of eight litter and sitting cases and making five round-trips per day, planners predicted their air-ambulance needs at twenty-one planes per division. Each squadron of air support would theoretically evacuate a division within a ten-hour period. However, since not all divisions would necessarily suffer the same percentages of wounded, planners estimated the need for two squadrons for each corps, or four squadrons for each army. This did not mean assigning squadrons to divisions or corps but attaching them instead to the chief surgeon at Aviation General Headquarters. In this manner, the chief surgeon could direct air-ambulance support as needed across the war theater.[38]

Planners designed the air-ambulance system to evacuate all but the slightly wounded from division and corps hospital stations to general hospitals. They considered the air ambulances impractical in advance of the division-hospital stations, which were normally situated four to six miles to the rear of the division front lines. Thus, the wounded were carried by ground transport from the collecting stations to suitable landing fields at the rear of a division for evacuation to general hospitals.

Given the probability that an insufficient number of landing fields would be available within any war zone, planners recommended combining division-hospital units at a single landing area. There, a combined medical team could triage the wounded into those slightly wounded, who could return to the front; those moderately wounded, who could be transported by motor ambulance to evacuation hospitals; and those more severely wounded, who would require immediate evacuation by air ambulance to general hospitals in the rear. Provided the system worked efficiently, injured men would arrive at the hospital station within two to four hours of being wounded and await further evacuation within one to three hours. In this manner, the wounded would receive surgical attention within a period of four to eight hours, thereby reducing significantly the problems of wound infection. In reviewing this overall action plan, strategists recognized the potential for reducing the number of evacuation hospitals, the possibility of consolidating divisional treatment stations and, at the same time, reducing the time between being at the battle line and receiving medical treatment.[39]

In general, medical planners anticipated that the air-ambulance system would reduce the scale of motor-ambulance transport between the division, the corps-hospital stations, and the evacuation hospitals and reduce as well the level of rail transportation required to move the wounded from evacuation hospitals to general hospitals. Overall, planners predicted that air-ambulance service would "probably reduce the present . . . army medical service by ten surgical hospitals, eight evacuation hospitals, two army medical regiments, and reduce the quantity of supplies carried in the army medical depot by one-third."[40]

ANGLES OF VISION

As planners down through the ages discovered, no single system for medical evacuation met the needs of the wounded under all conditions. Even the systems developed by Dr. Dominique-Jean Larrey and Dr. Jonathan Letterman had very different applications when faced with changes in strategy, tactics, logistics, and technology. Indeed, it would be a mistake—a caricature of history—to suggest that, in all the memoirs and histories of battles won and lost, there was a consistent relationship between the treatment and evacuation of the battle-wounded and the movements of armies and their various support systems. In fact, to follow the treatment of the wounded from one war—or from one battle—to another often gives the impression that everything learned in one was subsequently forgotten in the next. Planners, however rational their systems, inevitably faced the limitations created by events and by individuals whose skill or ignorance, rascality or virtue, were as varied as historians' views of the forces that produced events.

The limiting factors in a medical evacuation system varied from one war and one battle to another. For one country, at a given time and place, it might be the decision to attack or defend, of choosing objectives, deciding where and when to do battle, and assessing the costs of continued battle. For another, it might be the military's indifference to its wounded soldiers and the feeling that humanitarian acts, however laudable in principle, might jeopardize essential logistical support. At another time, the limiting factor might be interservice rivalry, for example, that between an established quartermaster's department and the aspirations of a budding medical department, which threaten a unified effort. Unwarranted competition, often the result of unenlightened personalities, interrupted orderly planning and frequently militated against a war effort. Other examples had more to do with the limitations of supply and transportation—port facilities; shortages of food or fodder; lack of railway networks, motor vehicles, or animals; and the impediments created by damaged or poorly constructed bridges, roads, and other communication links to and from the war zone. In yet other situations, the limiting factors related to questions about the ratio of service to combat troops; whether specialized units of soldiers should be organized and taken from units on the line and, if so, the problems of their training, morale, and efficiency; and whether civilians could or should be used to facilitate the evacuation of the wounded and the extent to which they should be supervised.

The evolution of medical evacuation systems followed both the experience of war and the impact of the industrial and transportation revolutions in each nation at war. The introduction of interchangeable parts, mass production, steam power, electricity, and railroads, as well as the utilization of the telegraph, the internal-combustion engine, and the airplane, had an impact on the ability of nations to wage war. Equally important, they all had an impact on the ability of nations to address the needs of their wounded in a timely and responsive way. And as these developments, along with those in metallurgy, chemistry, and physics, increased in pace in the late nineteenth and early twentieth centuries, similarities to problems of previous ages became more and more remote.

New weaponry changed the character and nature of combat, but without the revolution in transportation, the changes probably would have remained rudimentary. Increased mobility within and outside the war zone meant a difference in the way armies waged war. After centuries of reliance upon animals and human carrying parties, railroads made their first great impact, followed by motorized vehicles, and eventually air transport. The importance of these innovations cannot be minimized. Just as armies became increasingly tied to railroads, with the range of their military operations limited by their distance from railheads, so armies faced similar opportunities and constraints with respect to the evacuation of their wounded. Paradoxically, the very technology that spawned so much depersonalized violence also served to preserve and enhance life.

One should not, however, exaggerate the starkness of this underside of battle or the impersonal nature of war. Individual genius—in men like Larrey and Letterman, Dunant and Furley, Longmore and Hammond—became a powerful force in influencing events and the sometimes-misdirected or somnambulant actions of others. If there is indeed a connection between the activity of individuals and historical movement, it is found in the efforts of persons such as these who exercised a modicum of control, or at least self-expression, over the events that overpowered their generation. But it does not stop there, for to be effective, these same individuals had to cajole, force, intimidate, and convince others of the merits and reasonableness of their ideas. Basic to the success of any evacuation scheme was the art of asking the right questions—the art of the possible within the context of strategy, tactics, logistics, and existing technology. When we are able to combine the circumstances of war with the forcefulness and willpower of these individuals, we begin to understand the importance of the historical moment and its connectiveness in the life of nations. The value of a history of medical evacuation is to be judged not by the battles and campaigns alone but by the pertinent and cogent challenges made by various civilians and military professionals within the grimness of war, the cheapness of human life, and the paroxysms of national policy.

Notes
Selected Bibliography
Index

Notes

INTRODUCTION

1. Dr. Larrey quoted in George A. Otis, *A Report to the Surgeon General on the Transport of Sick and Wounded by Pack Animals* (Washington, D.C.: Government Printing Office, 1877), 2; W. E. Horner, "Ambulance," *American Cyclopedia of Practical Medicine and Surgery*, VI (1834), 338.

2. Thomas Longmore, "Ambulance," *Encyclopaedia Britannica: A Dictionary of Arts, Sciences and General Literature* (25 vols.; 9th ed.; Boston: Little, Brown, 1875–89), I, 665.

3. William G. Macpherson, "The Removal of Sick and Wounded from the Battlefield," *Journal of the Royal Army Medical Corps*, XII (1909), 82; Charles Smart, "Transportation of Wounded in War," *Proceedings*, Association of Military Surgeons of the United States, IV (1894), 42.

4. Paul Bronsart von Schellendorff, *The Duties of the General Staff* (London: W. A. H. Hare, 1895), 540.

1. BEGINNINGS OF A SYSTEM

1. Marcus Tullius Cicero, *Tusculan Disputations* (New York: Putnam, 1927), II, 16.38; John Scarborough, *Roman Medicine* (Ithaca, New York: Cornell University Press, 1969), 70–71.

2. W. E. Horner, "Ambulance," *American Cyclopedia of Practical Medicine and Surgery*, VI (1834), 339; Colonel Charles L. Heizmann, "Military Sanitation in the Sixteenth, Seventeenth and Eighteenth Centuries," *Annals of Medical History*, I (1917–18), 287; Fielding H. Garrison, "Notes on the History of Military Medicine," *Military Surgeon*, L (1922), 22–23, 326; Guido Majno, *The Healing Hand: Man and Wound in the Ancient World* (Cambridge, Massachusetts: Harvard University Press, 1975), 84, 382–85, 390, 393.

3. George A. Otis, *A Report to the Surgeon General on the Transport of Sick and Wounded by Pack Animals* (Washington, D.C.: Government Printing Office, 1877), 1–2.

4. Homer, *Iliad*, (London: Macmillan, 1886), V, 693; XIV, 429; XI, 517, 834.

5. N. Corbet Fletcher, *The St. John Ambulance Association: Its History, and Its Part in the Ambulance Movement* (London: St. John Ambulance Association, 1929), 5; Katherine T. Barkley, *The Ambulance: The Story of Emergency Transportation of Sick and Wounded Through the Centuries* (Hicksville, New York: Exposition Press, 1978), 14–15; E. T. Marten, "Modern Ambulances Have Developed from Rude Beginnings," *Modern Hospital*, XLII (1934), 43–46.

6. William K. R. Bedford and Richard Holbeche, *The Order of the Hospital of St. John of Jerusalem* (London: F. E. Robinson, 1902), 59–60; William K. R. Bedford, *Malta and the Knights Hospitallers* (London: Seeley, Service, 1903), 15, 17–18.

7. Garrison, "Notes on the History of Military Medicine," 319–21.

8. George Gask, *Essays in the History of Medicine* (London: Butterworth, 1950), 77–83, 99–100.

9. M. Mostyn Bird, *The Errand of Mercy: A History of Ambulance Work upon the Battlefield* (London: Hutchinson, 1913), 77–78.

10. Robert G. Richardson, *Larrey: Surgeon to Napoléon's Imperial Guard* (London: John Murray, 1974), 3; Garrison, "Notes on the History of Military Medicine," 160, 323–24.

11. Owen H. Wangensteen, Jacqueline Smith, and Sarah D. Wangensteen, "Some Highlights in the History of Amputation Reflecting Lessons in Wound Healing," *Bulletin of the History of Medicine*, XLI (1967), 97–131; Wallace B. Hamby, *Ambroise Paré: Surgeon of the Renaissance* (St. Louis, Missouri: Warren H. Green, 1967), 31–32; Joseph Francois Malgaigne, *Surgery and Ambroise Paré* (Norman: University of Oklahoma Press, 1965), 96, 239, 252, 261, 300, 321; Thomas Johnson (trans.), *The Workes of that Famous Chirurgion Ambrose Parey* (New York: Milford House, 1968 [1634]), 459–63.

12. Louis C. Duncan, *The Medical Department of the United States Army in the Civil War* (Gaithersburg, Maryland: Butternut Press, 1985), 380–81; Inspector General Sieur, "Tribulations of the Medical Corps of the French Army from its Origin to Our Own Times," *Military Surgeon*, LXIV (1929), 848–50; Garrison, "Notes on the History of Military Medicine," 453, 581.

13. Garrison, "Notes on the History of Military Medicine," 588, 593.

14. Oliver L. Spaulding, Jr., Hoffman Nickerson, and John W. Wright, *Warfare: A Study of Military Methods from the Earliest Times* (New York: Harcourt, Brace, 1925), 557–60, 566; Michael Howard, "Jomini and the Classical Tradition in Military Thought," in Michael Howard (ed.), *The Theory and Practice of War* (Bloomington: Indiana University Press, 1975), 5–20; Gunther E. Rothenberg, *The Art of Warfare in the Age of Napoleon* (London: B. T. Batsford, 1977), 14–17; Hew Strachan, *European Armies and the Conduct of War* (London: Allen and Unwin, 1983), 18.

15. Theodore A. Dodge, *Napoléon: A History of the Art of War, from the Beginning of the French Revolution to the End of the Eighteenth Century, with a Detailed Account of the Wars of the French Revolution* (4 vols.; Boston: Houghton Mifflin, 1904), I, 23.

16. Dodge, *Napoléon*, I, 24–28; II, 166–81, 313–16. J. Colin, *The Transformations of War* (Westport, Connecticut: Greenwood Press, 1977 [1912]), 27–28; Spaulding et al., *Warfare*, 570–72; Peter Paret, "Clausewitz and the Nineteenth Century," in Howard, *Theory and Practice of War*, 23–41; Rothenberg, *Art of Warfare*, 19–22.

17. Dominique-Jean Larrey, *Mémoires de chirurgie militaire, et campagnes* (4 vols.; Paris: J. Smith, 1812–17), I, 65–66, 150–58; Dominique-Jean Larrey, *Observations on Wounds, and Their Complications by Erysipelas, Gangrene and Tetanus, and on the Principal Diseases and Injuries of the Head, Ear and Eye* (Philadelphia: Key, Mielke and Biddle, 1832), 35.

18. Katherine T. Barkley, "The History of the Ambulance," *Proceedings*, International Congress of the History of Medicine (1974), 457; Heizmann, "Military Sanitation," 298–300; Thomas Longmore, *A Treatise on the Transport of Sick and Wounded Troops* (London: William Clowes, 1869), 27–28; James D. Edgar, "Baron Larrey, the Medical Officer," *Military Surgeon*, LIX (1926), 293.

19. James Henry Dible, *Napoléon's Surgeon* (London: Heinemann, 1970), 17–18.

20. Dr. Larrey quoted in Dible, *Napoléon's Surgeon*, 121; Charles Smart, "Transportation of Wounded in War," *Proceedings*, Association of Military Surgeons in the United States (1894), 24–25, 40; Richardson, *Larrey*, 23; Malgaigne, *Surgery and Ambroise Paré*, 252, 300.

21. Edgar, "Baron Larrey," 296; Owen H. Wangensteen, Sarah D. Wangensteen, and Charles F. Klinger, "Wound Management of Ambroise Paré and Dominique Larrey, Great French Military Surgeons of the 16th and 19th Centuries," *Bulletin of the History of Medicine*, XLVI (1972), 207–34; Dible, *Napoléon's Surgeon*, 120–23.

22. David M. Vess, *Medical Revolution in France, 1789–1796* (Gainesville: University Presses of Florida, 1975), 79–80; Smart, "Transportation of Wounded in War," 24–25; Albert A. Gore, "The Ambulance in War: Its Rise and Progress Amongst Civilized Nations," *Transactions*, Indian Medical Congress (1894), 347; Longmore, *Treatise*, 29–31; Bird, *Errand of Mercy*, 150–51.

23. Smart, "Transportation of Wounded in War," 25.

24. Smart, "Transportation of Wounded in War," 24–25; Surgeon Major George J. H. Evatt, *Ambulance Organization, Equipment, and Transport* (London: William Clowes, 1886), 6; Otis, *Report to the Surgeon General*, 2–3.

25. Venant A. L. Legouest, *Traité de chirurgie d'armée* (Paris: Baillière, 1863), 979; George Ballingall, *Outlines of Military Surgery* (Edinburgh: Adam and Charles Black, 1855), 116–17; Rothenberg, *Art of Warfare*, 228–31.

26. Gore, "The Ambulance in War," 347–48.

27. Gore, "The Ambulance in War," 347–48.

28. Garrison, "Notes on the History of Military Medicine," 702–3.

29. Fielding H. Garrison, "The Statistical Lessons of the Crimean War," *Military Surgeon*, XIV (1917), 459.

30. Quoted in Neil Cantlie, *A History of the Army Medical Department* (2 vols.; Edinburgh: Churchill Livingstone, 1974), II, 19, 6–9, 18, 46–47; John A. Shepherd, "The Surgeons in the Crimea," *Journal of the Royal College of Surgeons of*

Edinburgh, XVII (1972), 272–73; Longmore, *Treatise*, 36–37; Great Britain Army Medical Services, *Medical and Surgical History of the British Army Which Served in Turkey and the Crimea During the War Against Russia in the Years 1854–55–56* (2 vols.; London: Harrison, 1858), I, iii–iv; Siddha M. Mitra, *The Life and Letters of Sir John Hall* (New York: Longmans, Green, 1911), 520; John Fortescue and R. H. Beadon, *The Royal Army Service Corps: A History of Transport and Supply in the British Army* (2 vols.; Cambridge: Cambridge University Press, 1930–31), I, 150–51.

31. Cantlie, *A History of the Army Medical Department*, II, 12–13, 17.

32. Colonel Robert L. Reid, "The British Crimean Medical Disaster—Ineptness or Inevitability?" *Military Medicine*, CXL (1975), 422–23; Mitra, *Life and Letters of Sir John Hall*, 249–60, 311, 318–20, 331–33, 353–54; Longmore, *Treatise*, 38–39; Cantlie, *A History of the Army Medical Department*, II, 33–34.

33. Cantlie, *A History of the Army Medical Department*, II, 53.

34. William N. Boog Watson, "An Edinburgh Surgeon of the Crimean War—Patrick Heron Watson (1832–1907)," *Medical History*, X (1966), 169; A Lady Volunteer [Fanny Taylor], *Eastern Hospitals and English Nurses: The Narrative of Twelve Months' Experience in the Hospitals of Koulali and Scutari* (2 vols.; London: Hurst and Blackett, 1856), II, 14–21; George H. B. MacLeod, *War in the Crimea, with Remarks on the Treatment of Gunshot Wounds* (Philadelphia: Lippincott, 1862), 55–56.

35. Watson, "An Edinburgh Surgeon of the Crimean War," 168, 170; A Lady Volunteer, *Eastern Hospitals and English Nurses*, I, 100–101; Great Britain Army Medical Services, *Medical and Surgical History*, II, 171–77; Reid, "British Crimean Medical Disaster," 426.

36. Mitra, *Life and Letters of Sir John Hall*, 315; MacLeod, *War in the Crimea*, 323–25; John A. Shepherd, "The Smart of the Knife—Early Anaesthesia in the Services," *Journal of the Royal Army Medical Corps*, CXXXI (1985), 109–15; Cantlie, *A History of the Army Medical Department*, II, 13, 21, 191–92; George James Guthrie, *Commentaries on the Surgery of the War in Portugal, Spain, France, and the Netherlands, from the Battle of Rolica, in 1808, to That of Waterloo, in 1815: With Additions Relating to Those in the Crimea in 1854–55* (London: Henry Renshaw, 1855).

37. Shepherd, "Surgeons in the Crimea," 276–78; Reid, "British Crimean Medical Disaster," 420–21; Great Britain, Army Medical Services, *Medical and Surgical History*, II, 202–6; Cecil Woodham-Smith, *Florence Nightingale, 1820–1910* (London: Constable, 1950), 132, 184, 197, 203–5; Owen Wangensteen and Sarah D. Wangensteen, "Letters from a Surgeon in the Crimea," *Bulletin of the History of Medicine*, XLIII (1969), 376–79. Some thirty American surgeons served the Russian forces during the siege of Sebastopol. Most paid with their lives, dying from typhus and cholera. See E. Dvoichenko-Markov, "American Doctors in the Crimean War," *Journal of the History of Medicine*, IX (1954), 362–67; James A. Tobey, *The Medical Department of the Army: Its History, Activities and Organization* (Baltimore: Johns Hopkins University Press, 1927), 41.

38. Shepherd, "Surgeons in the Crimea," 283; John A. Shepherd, *Spencer Wells: The Life and Work of a Victorian Surgeon* (Edinburgh: E. and S. Livingstone, 1965), 31–32.

39. Mary C. Gillett, *The Army Medical Department 1775–1818* (Washington, D.C.: Government Printing Office, 1981), 22–28; Richard L. Blanco, "Medicine in the Continental Army, 1775–1781," *Bulletin*, New York Academy of Medicine, LVII (1981), 677–704; Philip Cash, *Medical Men at the Siege of Boston* (Philadelphia: American Philosophical Society, 1973), 16; Francis R. Packard, *History of Medicine in the United States* (2 vols.; New York: Hafner, 1963), I, 513–618.

40. Carl Jelenko, Judith B. Matthews, and John C. Matthews, "Emergency Medicine in Colonial America: Revolutionary War Casualties," *Annals of Emergency Medicine*, XI (1982), 73–76; H. L. Peterson, *The Book of the Continental Soldier* (Harrisburg, Pennsylvania: Promontory Press, 1968).

41. James A. Huston, *The Sinews of War: Army Logistics, 1775–1953* (Washington, D.C.: Office of the Chief of Military History, 1966), 99–100.

42. Garrison, "Notes on the History of Military Medicine," 701; Mary C. Gillett, *The Army Medical Department, 1818–1865* (Washington, D.C.: Center for Military History, 1987), 115–16, 132.

43. Richard Delafield, *Report of the Art of War in Europe in 1854, 1855 and 1856, by Major Richard Delafield, Corps of Engineers, From His Notes and Observations Made as a Member of a Military Commission to the Theatre of War in Europe, Under the Orders of the Honorable Jefferson Davis, Secretary of War* (Washington, D.C.: George W. Bowman, 1860), 2; Henry I. Bowditch, "Abuse of Army Ambulances," *Boston Medical and Surgical Journal*, LXVII (1862), 205; [Anonymous], "The Ambulance System," *North American Review*, XCVIII (1864), 74–75.

44. Bowditch, "Abuse of Army Ambulances," 205–6.

45. Gore, "The Ambulance in War," 349; Virginia R. Allen, "Medicine in the Union Armies," *Journal of the Oklahoma State Medical Association*, LXIV (1971), 460; Stewart Brooks, *Civil War Medicine* (Springfield, Illinois: Charles C. Thomas, 1966), 12, 16–20, 22–25, 111, 206–8; Julia C. Stimson, "Women Nurses with the Union Forces During the Civil War," *Military Surgeon*, LXII (1928), 2.

46. Casey Wood, "A Few Civil War Hospitals," *Military Surgeon*, XLII (1918), 539–40.

47. Mary A. Livermore, *My Story of the War: A Woman's Narrative of Four Years' Personal Experience as Nurse in the Union Army, and in Relief Work at Home, in Hospitals, Camps, and at the Front, During the War of the Rebellion* (Hartford, Connecticut: A. D. Worthington, 1889), 128–29; George W. Adams, *Doctors in Blue: The Medical History of the Union Army in the Civil War* (New York: Henry Schuman, 1952), 5–8; Francis A. Lord, *They Fought for the Union* (Harrisburg, Pennsylvania: Stackpole, 1960), 132; Gillett, *The American Medical Department, 1818–1865*, 161.

48. Jane T. Censer (ed.), *The Papers of Frederick Law Olmstead*, vol. 4, *Defending the Union: The Civil War and the U.S. Sanitary Commission, 1861–1863* (Baltimore: Johns Hopkins University Press, 1986), 15; Allen, "Medicine in the Union Armies," 462; Brooks, *Civil War Medicine*, 51, 60; Duncan, *The Medical Department*, 104; Charles J. Stillé, *History of the United States Sanitary Commission; Being the General Report of Its Work During the War of the Rebellion* (Philadelphia: Lippincott, 1866), 124; Livermore, *My Story of the War*, 133; United States

Sanitary Commission, *The Sanitary Commission of the United States Army: A Succinct Narrative of Its Works and Purposes* (New York: Arno Press, 1972 [1864]), 110.

49. Jacob G. Forman, *The Western Sanitary Commission. A Sketch of Its Origins, History, Labors for the Sick and Wounded of the Western Armies, and Aid Given to Freedmen and Union Refugees, With Incidents of Hospital Life* (St. Louis: R. P. Studley, 1864), 7; Censer, *The Papers of Frederick Law Olmstead*, 34, 52–53; Jack D. Key, "U.S. Army Department and Civil War Medicine," *Military Medicine*, CXXIII (1968), 189–91. The U.S. Christian Sanitary Commission was founded by Protestant ministers, the Young Men's Christian Association, and the American Tract Society on November 14, 1861, and relied upon unpaid volunteer labor. Unlike the secularly oriented U.S. Sanitary Commission and the Western Sanitary Commission, the Christian Sanitary Commission distributed evangelical religious tracts, wrote letters for soldiers, assisted in the dietary needs of hospital patients, and generally focused on the spiritual welfare of the soldier. Other organizations included the Women's Central Association of Relief and the Lint and Bandage Association.

50. Forman, *Western Sanitary Commission*, 12–15, 25–27, 110–15, 120.

51. Forman, *Western Sanitary Commission*, 62–63.

52. William Quentin Maxwell, *Lincoln's Fifth Wheel: The Political History of the United States Sanitary Commission* (New York: Longmans, Green, 1956), 8, 98; Western Sanitary Commission, *Report of the Western Sanitary Commission for the Year Ending June 1, 1863* (St. Louis: Western Sanitary Commission, 1863).

53. Smart, "Transportation of Wounded in War," 28.

54. Horner, "Ambulance," 339.

55. Horner, "Ambulance," 338–39.

56. Horner, "Ambulance," 341; Surgeon Major J. H. Porter, "Some Remarks on Aid to the Sick and Wounded in Time of War," *Lancet*, II (1876), 529–30.

57. Horner, "Ambulance," 339.

58. Smart, "Transportation of Wounded in War," 29–30.

59. Harvey E. Brown, *The Medical Department of the United States Army from 1775 to 1873* (Washington, D.C.: Surgeon General's Office, 1873), 212; Otis, *Report to the Surgeon General*, 2.

60. Smart, "Transportation of Wounded in War," 29; Duncan, *The Medical Department*, 38–39.

61. Duncan, *The Medical Department*, 17.

62. T. L. Rhoads, "Principles of Evacuation," *Military Surgeon*, LIV (1924), 284–85.

63. T. H. Squire, "Transportation of the Wounded from the Field of Battle," *Boston Medical and Surgical Journal*, LXXII (1861), 151–52.

64. Squire, "Transportation of the Wounded," 151–52.

65. Porter, "Some Remarks on Aid to the Sick and Wounded," 529–30.

66. Squire, "Transportation of the Wounded," 154–55; Otis, *Report to the Surgeon General*, 3; Longmore, *Treatise*, 1; Willis G. Diffenbaugh, "Military Surgery in the Civil War," *Military Medicine*, CXX (1965), 491–92; Adams, *Doctors in Blue*, 141.

67. Edward L. Munson, *The Principles of Sanitary Tactics: A Handbook on the Use of Medical Department Detachments and Organizations in Campaign* (Menasha, Wisconsin: George Banta, 1917), 15–17.

68. Quoted in United States Government, Surgeon General's Office, *The Medical and Surgical History of the War of the Rebellion (1861–65). Prepared, in Accordance with the Acts of Congress, Under the Direction of Surgeon General Joseph K. Barnes, United States Army* (3 parts in 6 vols.; Washington, D.C.: Government Printing Office, 1870–88), part III, vol. II, 932.

69. United States Government, Surgeon General's Office, *Medical and Surgical History*, part III, vol. II, 932.

70. Rhoads, "Principles of Evacuation," 285.

71. Bowditch, "Abuse of Army Ambulances," 204–5; Josiah Bartlett, "The Ambulance Service of the U.S. Army," *Transactions*, Medical Society of the State of New York, Albany (1863), 348; Duncan, *The Medical Department*, 78–81.

72. Bartlett, "Ambulance Service of the U.S. Army," 349.

73. Bartlett, "Ambulance Service of the U.S. Army," 350–51.

74. Bartlett, "Ambulance Service of the U.S. Army," 351–52; United States Government, Surgeon General's Office, *Medical and Surgical History*, part I, vol. I, 1–10.

75. Bartlett, "Ambulance Service of the U.S. Army," 348, 351.

76. Allen, "Medicine in the Union Armies," 461; Percy M. Ashburn, *A History of the Medical Department of the United States Army* (Boston: Houghton Mifflin, 1929), 75; John H. Brinton, *Personal Memoirs of John H. Brinton* (New York: Neal, 1914), 48, 171, 255; Alex Zeidenfelt, "The Embattled Surgeon, General William A. Hammond," *Civil War Times*, XVII (1978), 24–32; Louis C. Duncan, "The Strange Case of Surgeon General Hammond," *Military Surgeon*, LXIV (1929), 98–110, 252–62; Harvey C. Greisman, "William Hammond and His Enemies," *Medical Heritage*, II (1986), 322–31; William A. Hammond, *A Statement of the Causes Which Led to the Dismissal of Surgeon-General William A. Hammond from the Army* (New York: n.p., 1864); George W. Smith, *Medicines for the Union Army* (Madison, Wisconsin: American Institute of the History of Pharmacy, 1962), 3, 57–58; Gillett, *The Army Medical Department, 1818–1865*, 177–79, 201–3; Pascal James Imperato, "A History of the New York Medical Journal," *New York State Journal of Medicine*, LXXXIX (1989), 403–7.

77. United States Government, Surgeon General's Office, *Medical and Surgical History*, part III, vol. II, 933.

78. United States Government, Surgeon General's Office, *Medical and Surgical History*, part III, vol. II, 935–37.

79. Gillett, *The Army Medical Department, 1818–1865*, 190–91; Key, "U.S. Army Medical Department and Civil War Medicine," 188–90; Florence E. Oblensky, "Jonathan Letterman, 11 Dec. 1824–15 Mar. 1892," *Military Medicine* CXXXIII (1968), 312–15.

80. [Anonymous], "The Ambulance System," 86; Lucius L. Hopwood, "Duties of Ambulance Companies," *Military Surgeon*, XXXVII (1915), 234; Duncan, *The Medical Department*, 143–46; Ashburn, *A History of the Medical Department*, 88; Tobey, *The Medical Department of the Army*, 15–16; Rhoads, "Principles of Evacuation," 287, 289.

81. Barkley, "History of the Ambulance," 458; Rhoads, "Principles of Evacuation," 289; Gillett, *The Army Medical Department, 1818–1865*, 194; Brinton, *Personal Memoirs*, 215, 220.

82. Smart, "Transportation of Wounded in War," 33; Allen, "Medicine in the Union Armies," 461; Munson, *Principles of Sanitary Tactics*, 20–21.

83. United States Government, Surgeon General's Office, *Medical and Surgical History*, part III, vol. II, 905.

84. United States Government, Surgeon General's Office, *Medical and Surgical History*, part III, vol. II, 905.

85. David L. Nolan and David A. Pattillo, "The Army Medical Department and the Civil War: Historical Lessons for Current Medical Support," *Military Medicine*, CLIV (1989), 265–71; Duncan, *The Medical Department*, 117; Edward J. Stackpole, *Drama on the Rappahannock: The Fredericksburg Campaign* (Harrisburg, Pennsylvania: Military Service, 1957); Jonathan Letterman, *Medical Recollections of the Army of the Potomac* (New York: Appleton, 1866).

86. Hopwood, "Duties of Ambulance Companies," 234; Richard H. Shryock, *Medicine in America: Historical Essays* (Baltimore: Johns Hopkins University Press, 1966), 91.

87. Rhoads, "Principles of Evacuation," 291–92.

88. United States Government, Surgeon General's Office, *Medical and Surgical History*, part III, vol. I, 547; part III, vol. II, 901, 915. Allen, "Medicine in the Union Armies," 460–61; Smith, *Medicines for the Union Army*, 2; Michael Bradmore, "Some Aspects of the Confederate Medical Service," *Virginia Medical Monthly*, XCVIII (1971), 540; Adams, *Doctors in Blue*, 51, 119, 138.

89. Horace H. Cunningham, *Doctors in Gray: The Confederate Medical Service* (Baton Rouge: Louisiana State University Press, 1958), 116–22; Horace H. Cunningham, *Field Medical Services at the Battles of Manassas* (Athens: University of Georgia Press, 1968), 23–41, 69–91; Gordon W. Jones, "The Medical History of the Fredericksburg Campaign: Course and Significance," in Gert H. Brieger (ed.), *Theory and Practice in American Medicine* (New York: Science History, 1976), 186.

90. Thomas L. Livermore, *Numbers and Losses in the Civil War in America, 1861–1865* (Boston: Houghton, Mifflin, 1901), 2–5, 9, 47; Frederick Phistener, *Statistical Record of the Armies of the United States* (New York: Scribner, 1907), 70–71; James G. Randall and David Donald, *The Divided Union* (Boston; Little, Brown, 1961), 529–32.

91. [Anonymous], "The Ambulance System," 77.

2. EARLY AMBULANCE TECHNOLOGY

1. Richard Delafield, *Report of the Art of War in Europe in 1854, 1855 and 1856, by Major Richard Delafield, Corps of Engineers, From His Notes and Observations Made as a Member of a Military Commission to the Theatre of War in Europe, Under the Orders of the Honorable Jefferson Davis, Secretary of War* (Washington, D.C.: George W. Bowman, 1860), 73.

2. George J. H. Evatt, *Ambulance Organization, Equipment, and Transport* (London: William Clowes, 1886), 45; [Anonymous], "Dandies for Field Service,"

Indian Medical Gazette, V (1870), 256; Thomas Longmore, *A Treatise on the Transport of Sick and Wounded Troops* (London: William Clowes, 1869), 192–95; George Ballingall, *Outlines of Military Surgery* (Edinburgh: Adam and Charles Black, 1855), 118–19.

3. Longmore, *Treatise*, 97; F. H. Brett, "Camel Litters for the Conveyance of the Sick on the Line of March," *Indian Journal of Medicine and the Physical Sciences*, Calcutta, n.s. IV (1840), 150–51; Evatt, *Ambulance Organization*, 60; Ballingall, *Outlines of Military Surgery*, 120–21.

4. Delafield, *Report*, 73; [Anonymous], "The Ambulance System," *North American Review*, XCVIII (1864), 79–82.

5. George A. Otis, *A Report to the Surgeon General on the Transport of Sick and Wounded by Pack Animals* (Washington, D.C.: Government Printing Office, 1877), 6–7; United States Government, Surgeon General's Office, *The Medical and Surgical History of the War of the Rebellion (1861–65). Prepared, in Accordance with the Acts of Congress, Under the Direction of Surgeon General Joseph K. Barnes, United States Army* (3 parts in 6 vols.; Washington, D.C.: Government Printing Office, 1870–88), part III, vol. II, 927; Miller J. Stewart, *Moving the Wounded: Litters, Cacolets and Ambulance Wagons, U.S. Army, 1776–1876* (Fort Collins, Colorado: Old Army Press, 1979), 26.

6. Otis, *Report to the Surgeon General*, 9–10.

7. United States Government, Surgeon General's Office, *Medical and Surgical History*, part III, vol. II, 931.

8. United States Government, Surgeon General's Office, *Medical and Surgical History*, part III, vol. II, 931.

9. Ignaz Joseph Neudörfer, *Handbuch der Kriegschirurgie* (Leipzig: Vogel, 1864–67), 341; Otis, *Report to the Surgeon General*, 3; Albert A. Gore, "The Ambulance in War: Its Rise and Progress Amongst Civilized Nations," *Transactions*, Indian Medical Congress (1894), 350.

10. Valery Havard, "On Stretchers and Stretcher Drill," *Transactions*, Ninth International Medical Congress, Washington, D.C., II (1887), 56; United States Government, Surgeon General's Office, *Medical and Surgical History*, part III, vol. II, 923; T. H. Squire, "Transportation of the Wounded from the Field of Battle," *Boston Medical and Surgical Journal*, LXXII (1861), 152.

11. James P. Kimball, "Transportation of the Wounded in War," *Albany Medical Annals*, XIX (1898), 1195–96.

12. John H. Plumridge, *Hospital Ships and Ambulance Trains* (London: Seeley, Service, 1975), 86; George A. Otis, *A Report on a Plan for Transporting Wounded Soldiers by Railway in Time of War, With Descriptions of Various Methods Employed for This Purpose on Different Occasions* (Washington, D.C.: War Department, Surgeon General's Office, 1875), 27–28, 31.

13. G. H. Darwin, "The Different Methods of Lifting and Carrying the Sick and Injured," *Wood's Medical and Surgical Monographs*, VII (1890), 371, 374–75; J. H. Porter, "Some Remarks on Aid to the Sick and Wounded in Time of War," *Lancet*, II (1876), 529–30.

14. Thomas Longmore, "Report on the Fitness for Use in the British Service of a Wheeled Ambulance Transport Conveyance," *Report*, Army Medical Department, London, VII (1865), 505.

15. Dominique-Jean Larrey, *Mémoires de chirurgie militaire, et campagnes* (4 vols.; Paris: J. Smith, 1812–17), I, 168; Porter, "Some Remarks on Aid to the Sick and Wounded," 529–30; Alejandro Ross, "The Mexican Wheeled Stretcher for the Transport of Wounded on the Battlefield," *Military Surgeon*, XXIV (1909), 227–34.

16. Longmore, "Report on Fitness for Use," 505–14.

17. Longmore, "Report on Fitness for Use," 505, 509, 513–14; Ross, "Mexican Wheeled Stretcher," 227–34.

18. United States Government, Surgeon General's Office, *Medical and Surgical History*, part III, vol. II, 948; Charles Smart, "Transportation of Wounded in War," *Proceedings*, Association of Military Surgeons of the United States, IV (1894), 40; Katherine T. Barkley, "The History of the Ambulance," *Proceedings*, International Congress of the History of Medicine, London (1974), 458; Frank Hastings Hamilton, *A Practical Treatise on Military Surgery and Hygiene* (New York: Bailliere, 1861), 166–67; Longmore, *Treatise*, 358–59.

19. United States Government, Surgeon General's Office, *Medical and Surgical History*, part III, vol. II, 947–48.

20. United States Government, Surgeon General's Office, *Medical and Surgical History*, part III, vol. II, 949–50; Stewart, *Moving the Wounded*, 107–8; George W. Adair, "Wheeled Vehicles for the Transportation of Wounded," *Proceedings*, Association of Military Surgeons of the United States, IV (1894), 69–70.

21. J. D. Glennan, "The U.S. Army Ambulance—Its Advantages and Defects as Shown by Actual Service," *Proceedings*, Association of Military Surgeons of the United States, IV (1894), 69–70; James W. Wengert, "The 1878 Ambulance Board, Part I," *Military Collector and Historian*, XXXVII (1895), 8.

22. United States Government, Surgeon General's Office, *Medical and Surgical History*, part III, vol. II, 955–56.

23. Stewart, *Moving the Wounded*, 36; Horace H. Cunningham, *Doctors in Gray: The Confederate Medical Service* (Baton Rouge: Louisiana State University Press, 1958), 115–20.

24. Wengert, "1878 Ambulance Board, Part I," 22; James W. Wengert, "The 1878 Ambulance Board, Part II," *Military Collector and Historian*, XXXVII (1986), 50–67; Smart, "Transportation of Wounded in War," 70.

25. Plumridge, *Hospital Ships and Ambulance Trains*, 24–28.

26. Smart, "Transportation of Wounded in War," 71.

27. Jane T. Censer (ed.), *The Papers of Frederick Law Olmstead*, vol. 4, *Defending the Union: The Civil War and the U.S. Sanitary Commission, 1861–1863* (Baltimore: Johns Hopkins University Press, 1986), 28–30, 310, 330–31, 404–5.

28. United States Government, Surgeon General's Office, *Medical and Surgical History*, part III, vol. II, 976, 981; Jacob G. Forman, *The Western Sanitary Commission. A Sketch of Its Origins, History, Labors for the Sick and Wounded of the Western Armies, and Aid Given to Freedmen and Union Refugees, With Incidents of Hospital Life* (St. Louis: R. P. Studley, 1864), 106.

29. Barkley, "History of the Ambulance," 458.

30. Quoted in United States Government, Surgeon General's Office, *Medical and Surgical History*, part III, vol. II, 973; Percy M. Ashburn, *A History of the Medical Department of the United States* (Boston: Houghton Mifflin, 1929), 80.

31. United States Government, Surgeon General's Office, *Medical and Surgical History*, part III, vol. II, 986.

32. Otis, *Report on a Plan*, 4.

33. Cyril B. Falls, *The Art of War: From the Age of Napoléon to the Present Day* (New York: Oxford University Press, 1961), 66–67.

34. Otis, *Report on a Plan*, 5; Plumridge, *Hospital Ships and Ambulance Trains*, 83; Smart, "Transportation of Wounded in War," 44; Evatt, *Ambulance Organization*, 89–90; Russell F. Weigley, *History of the United States Army* (New York: Macmillan, 1967), 222–25; John E. Ransom, "The Development of Ambulance Service in the Armies of Great Britain, the United States and Other Countries," *Ciba Symposia*, VIII (1946), 554–59; Mary C. Gillett, *The Army Medical Department, 1818–1865* (Washington, D.C.: Center for Military History, 1987), 293–95.

35. Louis W. Read, "Railway Transportation of Sick and Wounded," *Proceedings*, Association of Military Surgeons of the United States, IV (1894), 84–90.

36. Ashburn, *A History of the Medical Department*, 81.

37. Otis, *Report on a Plan*, 11–12; United States Government, Surgeon General's Office, *Medical and Surgical History*, appendix to part I, 289; Read, "Railway Transportation of Sick and Wounded," 87.

38. Otis, *Report on a Plan*, 7–8; Read, "Railway Transportation of Sick and Wounded," 86.

39. Otis, *Report on a Plan*, 16–17; DeForest Willard, *Ambulance Service in Philadelphia* (Philadelphia: n.p., 1883), 19–20; United States Government, Surgeon General's Office, *Medical and Surgical History*, part III, vol. II, chapter 15.

40. Hamilton, *Practical Treatise*, 168.

41. Henry McElderry, *Descriptions of the Models of Hospital Cars, From the U.S. Army Medical Museum, Washington, D.C.* (New Orleans: The World's Industrial and Cotton Centennial Exposition, 1884–85), 4–5; Otis, *Report on a Plan*, 13, 16–17; United States Government, *International Exhibition of 1876. Hospital of Medical Department, United States Army. Description of the Models of Hospital Cars* (Washington, D.C.: Government Printing Office, 1876), 4–5; Harvey E. Brown, *The Medical Department of the United States Army From 1775 to 1873* (Washington, D.C.: Surgeon General's Office, 1873), 236.

42. Otis, *Report on a Plan*, 7.

43. Otis, *Report on a Plan*, 22; Charles J. Stillé, *History of the United States Sanitary Commission; Being the General Report of Its Work During the War of the Rebellion* (Philadelphia: Lippincott, 1866), 163–65.

44. Quoted in John Van R. Hoff, "The Travois—A New Sanitary Appliance in the First Line of Battlefield Assistance," *Proceedings*, Association of Military Surgeons of the United States, IV (1894), 89; Otis, *Report on a Plan*, 23; John J. Chisolm, *A Manual of Military Surgery, for the Use of Surgeons in the Confederate Army* (Charleston: Evans and Cogswell, 1861), chapter 3, 99–106; Cunningham, *Doctors in Gray*, 122–23.

45. Quoted in Willard, *Ambulance Service in Philadelphia*, 17; Hoff, "The Travois," 89.

46. Francis Parkman, *History of the Conspiracy of Pontiac, and the War of the North American Tribes Against the English Colonies After the Conquest of Canada*

(Boston: Little, Brown, 1851), 601; Francis Parkman, *California and Oregon Trail: Being Sketches of Prairie and Rocky Mountain Life* (New York: Putnam, 1849), 165; Paul Allen, *History of the Expedition Under the Command of Captains Lewis and Clark, to the Sources of the Missouri, Thence Across the Rocky Mountains and Down the River Columbia to the Pacific Ocean. Performed During the Years 1804–5–6, by Order of the Government of the United States* (Philadelphia: Bradford and Inskeep, 1817), II, 381; Drake W. Will, "The Medical and Surgical Practice of the Lewis and Clark Expedition," in Gert H. Brieger (ed.), *Theory and Practice in American Medicine* (New York: Science History Publications, 1976), 124–48; Otis, *Report to the Surgeon General*, 11.

47. William B. Lord and Thomas Baines, *Shifts and Expedients of Camp Life, Travel, and Exploration* (London: Sheldon, 1871); Charles A. Gordon, *Army Hygiene* (London: Churchill, 1866), 217; Otis, *Report to the Surgeon General*, 4–5; Randolph B. Marcy, *The Prairie Traveler. A Hand-book for Overland Expeditions* (New York: Harper, 1859), 150–54.

48. Otis, *Report to the Surgeon General*, 5–6; Marcia Brace Kimball, *A Soldier-Doctor of Our Army: James P. Kimball* (Boston: Houghton Mifflin, 1917), 27–93.

49. Hoff, "The Travois," 73–75, 78–82; Stewart, *Moving the Wounded*, 63–64.

50. Otis, *Report to the Surgeon General*, 18–20; William E. Strong, *A Trip to the Yellowstone National Park, in July, August, and September, 1875* (Washington, D.C.: n.p., 1876), 75; Charles Albert Sewall, "The New Extemporaneous Litter, Copied After the Mojave Indian Method of Carrying the Wounded," *Medical Record*, XXVIII (1890), 461–62.

51. Otis, *Report to the Surgeon General*, 23.

52. Otis, *Report to the Surgeon General*, 15–16.

53. Otis, *Report to the Surgeon General*, 11.

54. Otis, *Report to the Surgeon General*, 13.

55. United States Government, Surgeon General's Office, *Medical and Surgical History*, part III, vol. II, 917–19.

56. Otis, *Report to the Surgeon General*, 19.

57. David L. Huntington and George A. Otis, *Hospital of Medical Department, United States Army. No. 6. Description of the U.S. Army Medical Transport Cart, Model of 1876* (Philadelphia: International Exhibition, 1876), 3–16.

3. A WORLD IN TRANSITION

1. S. Morganstern, "Henry Dunant and the Red Cross," *Bulletin*, New York Academy of Medicine, LV (1979), 949–56; E. T. Marten, "Modern Ambulances Have Developed from Rude Beginnings," *Modern Hospital*, XLII (1934), 457; Jean-Henry Dunant, *Un Souvenir de Solférino* (Geneve: J. Cherbuliez, 1862); Martin Gumpert, *Dunant: The Story of the Red Cross* (New York: Oxford University Press, 1938), 63; Violet K. Libby, *Henry Dunant: Prophet of Peace* (New York: Pagent Press, 1964).

2. Marten, "Modern Ambulances," 457.

3. Gumpert, *Dunant*, 171; Katherine T. Barkley, *The Ambulance: The Story of Emergency Transportation of Sick and Wounded Through the Centuries* (Hicksville,

New York: Exposition Press, 1978), 35; Myles Standish, "The Organization, Equipment, Instruction and Drill of the Ambulance Corps (Hospital Corps) of the Massachusetts Volunteer Militia," *Proceedings*, Association of Military Surgeons of the United States, IV (1894), 54.

4. Neil Cantlie, *A History of the Army Medical Department* (2 vols.; Edinburgh: Churchill Livingstone, 1974), II, 271–72.

5. Clara Barton, *The Red Cross: A History of This Remarkable Movement in the Interest of Humanity* (Washington, D.C.: American National Red Cross, 1898), 23–24; George J. H. Evatt, *Ambulance Organization, Equipment, and Transport* (London: William Clowes, 1886), 16; [Anonymous], "What Is Done for the Wounded; How They Are Collected at the Front and Transferred to the Permanent Hospitals," *Scientific American*, LXXXI (1916), 1196; John Furley, "The Convention of Geneva, and the Care of the Sick and Wounded in War," *Journal of the Royal United Service Institution*, XL (1896), 1215.

6. William G. Macpherson, "The Removal of Sick and Wounded from the Battlefield," *Journal of the Royal Army Medical Corps*, XII (1909), 87–88.

7. Albert A. Gore, "The Ambulance in War: Its Rise and Progress Amongst Civilized Nations," *Transactions*, Indian Medical Congress (1894), 347; Fielding H. Garrison, "Notes on the History of Military Medicine," *Military Surgeon*, L (1922), 712.

8. Furley, "Convention of Geneva," 1218. John Furley was director of ambulances during the Franco-Prussian War, was director of the flying ambulance attached to Marshal Marie-Maurice de MacMahon's army against the commune in 1871, and served in the Carlists' War and at Montenegro in 1877.

9. Furley, "Convention of Geneva," 1219; John Clifford, *For the Service of Mankind: Furley, Lechmere and Duncan, St. John Ambulance Founders* (London: Robert Hale, 1971), 19–30, 99–101.

10. Gumpert, *Dunant*, 248–60.

11. Furley, "Convention of Geneva," 1221.

12. Valentine A. J. Swain, "Franco-Prussian War 1870–1871: Voluntary Aid for the Wounded and Sick," *British Medical Journal*, III (1870), 511.

13. W. G. N. Manley and G. W. McNalty, "Reports on the Construction and Equipment of the British Service Ambulance Wagon," *Report of the British National Society To Aid Sick and Wounded in War, Franco-German War* (London: n.p., 1871), 178–83.

14. N. Corbet Fletcher, *The St. John Ambulance Association: Its History, and Its Part in the Ambulance Movement* (London: St. John Ambulance Association, 1929), 10; Sir John Furley, *In Peace and War: Autobiographical Sketches* (London: Smith, Elder, 1905), 45; William MacCormac, *Notes and Recollections of an Ambulance Surgeon, Being an Account of Work Done Under the Red Cross During the Campaign of 1870* (London: J. and A. Churchill, 1871), 19–21.

15. Archibald Forbes, *My Experiences of the War Between France and Germany* (2 vols.; London: Hurst and Blackett, 1871), I, 250–51; Swain, "Franco-Prussian War," 513; Furley, *In Peace and War*, 33–36, 50–51.

16. H. E. R. James, "Adaptation of Motor Omnibus and Scotch Haycart for Carriage of Wounded Men," *Journal of the Royal Army Medical Corps*, XV (1910), 69–77.

17. George A. Otis, *A Report to the Surgeon General on the Transport of Sick and Wounded by Pack Animals* (Washington, D.C.: Government Printing Office, 1877), 2; Gore, "The Ambulance in War," 352.

18. Swain, "Franco-Prussian War," 512.

19. George A. Otis, *A Report on a Plan for Transporting Wounded Soldiers by Railway in Time of War, with Descriptions of Various Methods Employed for This Purpose on Different Occasions* (Washington, D.C.: War Department, Surgeon General's Office, 1875), 39–40.

20. Otis, *Report on a Plan*, 36; A. Zavodovsky, *Transport spécial des malades et des Blessés en temps de guerre, par voies ferrées* (Saint Petersburg: n.p., 1874).

21. Otis, *Report on a Plan*, 37; Evatt, *Ambulance Organization*, 97–100; John H. Plumridge, *Hospital Ships and Ambulance Trains* (London: Seeley, Service, 1975), 87–88.

22. Quoted in Michael Howard, *The Franco-Prussian War: The German Invasion of France, 1870–1871* (London: Methuen, 1967), 2–3; Edwin A. Pratt, *The Rise of Rail Power in War and Conquest, 1833–1914* (London: P. S. King, 1915), 2–3; Edward M. Earle, *Makers of Modern Strategy: Military Thought from Machiavelli to Hitler* (Princeton, New Jersey: Princeton, University Press, 1943), 148–52.

23. F. L. Pleadwell, "British Ambulance Trains," *Military Surgeon*, XLVI (1920), 52.

24. H. E. R. James and C. E. Pollock, "Notes on the Conveyance of Sick and Wounded by Rail, with Special Reference to Improvised Methods," *Journal of the Royal Army Medical Corps*, XV (1910), 276–77.

25. Macpherson, "Removal of Sick and Wounded," 85–86, 92.

26. Furley, "Convention of Geneva," 1221.

27. Furley, "Convention of Geneva," 1223–24.

28. Charles S. Ryan, *Under the Red Crescent: Adventures of an English Surgeon with the Turkish Army at Plevna and Erzerum, 1877–1878* (New York: Scribner, 1897), 128–29.

29. Ryan, *Under the Red Crescent*, 136.

30. Charles Smart, "Transportation of Wounded in War," *Proceedings*, Association of Military Surgeons of the United States, IV (1894), 38.

31. Cantlie, *A History of the Army Medical Department*, II, 196–232.

32. Cantlie, *A History of the Army Medical Department*, II, 232–34, 274–79.

33. Cantlie, *A History of the Army Medical Department*, II, 280–81.

34. Hew Strachan, *European Armies and the Conduct of War* (London: Allen and Unwin, 1983), 76–77; Charles Edward Callwell, *Small Wars. Their Principles and Practice* (3d ed.; London: Trowbridge and Esher, 1976 [1906]).

35. G. B. Carter, "Ambulance Work in Hill Warfare from Front to Base," *Journal of the Royal Army Medical Corps*, V (1905), 509–512; P. C. Gabbett, "Transport and Treatment of Sick and Wounded on the Lines of Communication in Indian Frontier Warfare," *Indian Medical Gazette*, Calcutta, XXXIII (1898), 433–35.

36. [Anonymous], "The Camel Ambulance," *Proceedings*, Association of Military Surgeons of the United States, XIX (1906), 77–78.

37. R. Vacy Ash, "Transport of Sick and Wounded in Uncivilized Countries, Bearing Especially on the Late Kaffir Campaigns," *Transactions*, Seventh International Medical Congress, II (1881), 501–2; M. Mostyn Bird, *The Errand of Mercy: A History of Ambulance Work upon the Battlefield* (London: Hutchinson, 1913), 284–89.

38. Ash, "Transport of Sick and Wounded in Uncivilized Countries," 503–4; T. P. Jones, "A Report upon the Transport of the Sick and Wounded in the Field," *Journal of the Royal Army Medical Corps*, III (1904), 582–83.

39. Carter, "Ambulance Work in Hill Warfare," 512, 515; R. F. Tobin, "A Memoir of the Late Lieutenant-Colonel Charles Dalton, R.A.M.C.," *Journal of the Royal Army Medical Corps*, XXVIV (1915), 64–94.

40. Jones, "Report upon the Transport of Sick and Wounded," 580–81.

41. A. R. Tweedie, "Ambulance Wagon. Mark I (Light)," *Journal of the Royal Army Medical Corps*, XV (1910), 695–701.

42. Hew Strachan, *From Waterloo to Balaclava: Tactics, Technology, and the British Army, 1815–1854* (Cambridge: Cambridge University Press, 1985), 55–91.

43. W. Y. Carman, *A History of Firearms from Earliest Times to 1914* (New York: St. Martin's Press, 1955), 122–23, 130.

44. Quoted in T. F. S. Caverhill, "Description of Ambulance for the Mounted Service," *British Medical Journal*, I (1900), 67; Brian Bond, "Doctrine and Training in the British Cavalry, 1870–1914," in Michael Howard (ed.), *The Theory and Practice of War* (Bloomington: Indiana University Press, 1975), 97–99.

45. Howard, *Theory and Practice of War*, 101, 104–5, 115; Douglas Haig, *Cavalry Studies: Strategical and Tactical* (London: H. Rees, 1907); Frederick A. J. Bernhardi, *Cavalry in Future Wars* (New York: Dutton, 1906); H. C. B. Rogers, *The Mounted Troops of the British Army, 1066–1945* (London: Seeley Service, 1959); Frederick N. Maude, *Cavalry Versus Infantry* (Kansas City, Missouri: Hudson-Kimberly, 1896); Erskine Childers, *War and the Arme Blanche* (London: E. Arnold, 1910); Callwell, *Small Wars*, 401–24; Strachan, *European Armies*, 84–85.

46. Quoted in Caverhill, "Description of Ambulance for the Mounted Service," 67; T. F. S. Caverhill, "Cavalry Ambulance Service," *British Medical Journal*, II (1900), 625–26.

47. Gore, "The Ambulance in War," 355.

48. H. G. Hathaway, "Ambulance for Mounted Troops," *Proceedings*, Association of Military Surgeons of the United States, XIII (1903), 134–40; H. G. Hathaway, "The Disposal of the Wounded of Strategical Cavalry," *Journal of the Royal Army Medical Corps*, XV (1910), 308–10.

49. Jones, "Report upon the Transport of Sick and Wounded," 577.

50. Jerry M. Cooper, "The Wisconsin National Guard in the Milwaukee Riots of 1866," in Peter Karsten (ed.), *The Military in America: From the Colonial Era to the Present* (New York: Free Press, 1980), 209–25; Jerry M. Cooper, "The Army's Search for a Mission, 1865–1890," in Kenneth J. Hagan and William R. Roberts (eds.), *Against All Enemies: Interpretations of American Military History from Colonial Times to the Present* (Westport, Connecticut: Greenwood Press, 1986), 173–95; William A. Ganoe, *The History of the United States Army* (Ashton, Maryland: Eric Lundberg, 1964) 298–354; Edward M. Coffman, *The Old Army:*

A Portrait of the American Army in Peacetime, 1784–1898 (New York: Oxford University Press, 1986), 215–16.

51. Russell F. Weigley, *The American Way of War: A History of United States Military Strategy and Policy* (New York: Macmillan, 1973), 153–63.

52. Weigley, *The American Way of War*, 169; Emanual R. Lewis, *Seacoast Fortifications of the United States: An Introductory History* (Washington, D.C.: Smithsonian Institute Press, 1970); Graham A. Cosmas, *An Army for Empire: The United States Army in the Spanish-American War* (Columbia: University of Missouri Press, 1971), 7, 84, 86; Ganoe, *History of the United States Army*, 355–96.

53. Allan R. Millett and Peter Maslowski, *For the Common Defense: A Military History of the United States of America* (New York: Free Press, 1984), 256–64; Stephen E. Ambrose, *Upton and the Army* (Baton Rouge: Louisiana State University Press, 1964); Peter Karsten, *The Naval Aristocracy: The Golden Age of Annapolis and the Emergence of Modern American Navalism* (New York: Free Press, 1972); Albert Gleaves, *Life and Letters of Rear Admiral Stephen B. Luce* (New York: Putnam, 1925); Peter Karsten, "Armed Progressives: The Military Reorganizes for the American Century," in Peter Karsten, *The Military in America*, 239–74; Russell F. Weigley, *History of the United States Army* (New York: Macmillan, 1967), 233–64.

54. Charles Smart, "First Aid to the Injured, from the Army Stand-Point," *Medical Record*, XLIV (1893), 71.

55. Standish, "Organization, Equipment, Instruction and Drill," 54–55; Smart, "Transportation of Wounded in War," 33–36; Smart, "First Aid to the Injured," 71.

56. Nicholas Senn, *Medico-Surgical Aspects of the Spanish-American War* (Chicago: American Medical Association Press, 1900), 55–57; Nicholas Senn, *War Correspondence* (Chicago: American Medical Association Press, 1899), 41–45.

57. Senn, *War Correspondence*, 72.

58. Percy M. Ashburn, *A History of the Medical Department of the United States Army* (Boston: Houghton Mifflin, 1929), 157, 174–75; James A. Tobey, *The Medical Department of the Army: Its History, Activities and Organization* (Baltimore: Johns Hopkins University Press, 1927), 25–27; Senn, *Medico-Surgical Aspects*, 58; David F. Trask, *The War with Spain in 1898* (New York: Macmillan, 1981), 295.

59. John M. Gibson, *Soldier in White: The Life of General George Miller Sternberg* (Durham, North Carolina: Duke University Press, 1958), 188; Trask, *The War with Spain in 1898*, 160–61.

60. Gibson, *Soldier in White*, 189; United States Government, War Department, "Report of Colonel Charles R. Greenleaf, Chief Surgeon, 24 August, 1898," *Annual Reports of the War Department for the Fiscal Year Ended June 30, 1898* (Washington, D.C.: Government Printing Office, 1898), 73.

61. Gibson, *Soldier in White*, 191–92; Cosmas, *An Army for Empire*, 249–50; Senn, *War Correspondence*, 55–60.

62. Herbert R. Collins, "Red Cross Ambulance of 1898," *United States National Museum Bulletin*, No. 241 (Washington, D.C.: Smithsonian Institute, 1965), 167.

63. Quoted in William E. Barton, *The Life of Clara Barton, Founder of the American Red Cross* (2 vols.; New York: AMS Press, 1969), I, 4; Katherine T. Barkley, "The History of the Ambulance," *Proceedings*, International Congress of the History of Medicine, London (1974), 460; Collins, "Red Cross Ambulance of 1898," 170–73; Barton, *The Red Cross: A History*, 446–47.

64. Gibson, *Soldier in White*, 209–10, 212; Cosmas, *An Army for Empire*, 282–98; Margaret Leech, *In the Days of McKinley* (New York: Harper, 1959), 313–14.

65. George M. Sternberg, *Sanitary Lessons of the War, and Other Papers* (Washington, D.C.: Bryon S. Adams, 1912), 15.

66. Brian McAllister Linn, *The U.S. Army and Counterinsurgency in the Philippine War, 1899–1902* (Chapel Hill: University of North Carolina Press, 1989), 2; William T. Sexton, *Soldiers in the Sun: An Adventure in Imperialism* (Harrisburg, Pennsylvania: Military Services, 1939); N. N. Freeman, *A Soldier in the Philippines* (New York: F. Tennyson Neely, 1901); Frederick Funston, *Memories of Two Wars: Cuban and Philippine Experiences* (New York: Scribner, 1914); Millett and Maslowski, *For the Common Defense*, 290–97; Stewart C. Miller, *"Benevolent Assimilation": The American Conquest of the Philippines, 1899–1903* (New Haven, Connecticut: Yale University Press, 1982); Joseph L. Schott, *The Ordeal of Samar* (Indianapolis: Bobbs-Merrill, 1964).

67. United States Government, War Department, "Report of the Surgeon General," *Annual Reports of the War Department for the Fiscal Year Ended June 30, 1900* (Washington, D.C.: Government Printing Office, 1900), 633.

68. United States Government, War Department, "Report of the Surgeon General," (1900), 652.

69. Mary C. Gillett, "Medical Care and Evacuation during the Philippine Insurrection, 1899–1901," *Journal of the History of Medicine*, XLII (1987), 184.

70. John Morgan Gates, *Schoolbooks and Krags: The United States Army in the Philippines, 1898–1902* (Westport, Connecticut: Greenwood Press, 1973), 96.

71. United States Government, War Department, "Report of the Surgeon General," (1900), 669.

72. United States Government, War Department, "Report of the Surgeon General," (1900), 604.

73. William J. Lyster, "The Army Surgeon in the Philippines," *Journal of the American Medical Association*, XXXVI (1901), 32.

74. Quoted in George M. Sternberg, "Medical and Sanitary History of the Troops in the Philippines," *Philadelphia Medical Journal*, VI (1900), 829–30.

75. Lyster, "Army Surgeon in the Philippines," 30.

76. Sternberg, "Medical and Sanitary History of Troops in the Philippines," 826.

77. Gillett, "Medical Care and Evacuation," 177.

78. United States Government, War Department, "Report of the Surgeon General," (1900), 615.

79. United States Government, War Department, "Report of the Surgeon General," (1900), 615.

4. OLD AND NEW THINKING

1. James P. Kimball, "Transportation of the Wounded in War," *Albany Medical Annals*, XIX (1898), 202; George W. Adair, "Wheeled Vehicles for the Transportation of Wounded," *Proceedings*, Association of Military Surgeons of the United States, VI (1896), 146–51.

2. W. J. B., "Sanitary Appliances at the Centennial," *Sanitarian*, III (1876), 459–60.

3. Gore, "The Ambulance in War: Its Rise and Progress Amongst Civilized Nations," *Transactions*, Indian Medical Congress (1894), 353, 355; J. H. Ford, "Notes on Organization and Equipment for Evacuation of the Wounded," *Military Surgeon*, XXXI (1912), 685.

4. C. H. Melville, "Casualties in Modern War from the Point of View of an Ambulance Surgeon," *Transactions*, First Indian Medical Congress, 1894 (1895), 350; Kimball, "Transportation of the Wounded in War," 196–97.

5. Gore, "The Ambulance in War," 355; Ford, "Notes on Organization and Equipment," 680; [Anonymous], "The H. L. Getz Improved Bicycle Ambulance and Hand-Stretcher," *Railway Surgeon*, V (1898–99), 180–81; Kimball, "Transportation of the Wounded in War," 199–200.

6. Kimball, "Transportation of the Wounded in War," 200–201.

7. Valery Havard, "Litter and Ambulance Transportation," *Proceedings*, Association of Military Surgeons of the United States, IV (1894), 46; T. P. Jones, "A Report upon the Transport of the Sick and Wounded in the Field," *Journal of the Royal Army Medical Corps*, III (1904), 580.

8. Havard, "Litter and Ambulance Transportation," 48, 50.

9. William G. Macpherson, "The Removal of Sick and Wounded from the Battlefield," *Journal of the Royal Army Medical Corps*, XII (1909), 90–91; Ford, "Notes on Organization and Equipment," 685; M. Mostyn Bird, *The Errand of Mercy: A History of Ambulance Work upon the Battlefield* (London: Hutchinson, 1913), 297.

10. George M. Dupuy, *The Stretcher Bearer: A Companion to the R.A.M.C. Training Book, Illustrating the Stretcher Bearer Drill and the Handling and Carrying of Wounded* (London: Oxford University Press, 1915), 44–63; J. J. de Zouche Marshall, *Stretcher Drill* (London: J. and A. Churchill, 1904), 1–35.

11. Charles Smart, "First Aid to the Injured, from the Army Stand-Point," *Medical Record*, XLIV (1893), 73.

12. Smart, "First Aid to the Injured," 73.

13. Nicholas Senn, *Medico-Surgical Aspects of the Spanish-American War* (Chicago: American Medical Association Press, 1900), 298–300; George M. Sternberg, *Sanitary Lessons of the War, and Other Papers* (Washington, D.C.: Bryon S. Adams, 1912), 1–8; M. W. Ireland (ed.), *The Medical Department of the United States Army in the World War*, vol. XI, *Surgery* (Washington, D.C.: Government Printing Office, 1927), xxx–xxxi.

14. Smart, "First Aid to the Injured," 73.

15. Smart, "First Aid to the Injured," 73–74; Gore, "The Ambulance in War," 356.

16. Macpherson, "Removal of Sick and Wounded," 79–80.

17. Ford, "Notes on Organization and Equipment," 671.

18. Macpherson, "Removal of Sick and Wounded," 84–85.

19. Jay Luvaas, "European Military Thought and Doctrine, 1870–1914," in Michael Howard (ed.), *The Theory and Practice of War* (Bloomington: Indiana University Press 1975), 71–93.

20. Michael Howard, *The Franco-Prussian War: The German Invasion of France, 1870--871* (London: Methuen, 1967), 5–6; Charles B. Brackenbury, *European Armaments in 1867* (London: Chapman and Hall, 1867); J. Colin, *The Transformations of War* (Westport, Connecticut: Greenwood Press, 1977 [1912]), 29–31; F. Maurice, *The System of Field Manoeuvres Best Adapted for Enabling Our Troops To Meet a Continental Army* (2d ed.; London: William Blackwood, 1872), 11–12.

21. Howard, *Franco-Prussian War*, 35; Archibald Forbes, *My Experiences of the War Between France and Germany* (2 vols.; London: Hurst and Blackett, 1871), I, 209–11; Gore, "The Ambulance in War," 357; W. Y. Carman, *A History of Firearms from Earliest Times to 1914* (New York: St. Martin's Press, 1955), 121.

22. James C. Beyer (ed.), *Wound Ballistics* (Washington, D.C.: Department of the Army, 1962), 127–31; Louis A. LaGarde, *Gunshot Injuries: How They Are Inflicted, Their Complications and Treatment* (2d ed.; New York: William Wood, 1916); W. F. Stevenson, *Wounds in War* (New York: William Wood, 1898).

23. Beyer, *Wound Ballistics*, 137–41; L. B. Wilson, "Dispersion of Bullet Energy in Relation to Wound Effects," *Military Surgeon*, XLIX (1921), 241–51.

24. Fielding H. Garrison, "Notes on the History of Military Medicine," *Military Surgeon*, L (1922), 712.

25. Cyril B. Falls, *The Art of War: From the Age of Napoléon to the Present Day* (New York: Oxford University Press, 1961), 64–66.

26. Paul F. Straub, *Medical Service in Campaign: A Handbook for Medical Officers in the Field* (Philadelphia: P. Blakiston, 1910), 28.

27. Straub, *Medical Service in Campaign*, 29.

28. Lucius L. Hopwood, "Duties of Ambulance Companies," *Military Surgeon*, XXXVII (1915), 229.

29. William G. Macpherson (ed.), *History of the Great War Based on Official Documents*, vol. I, *Medical Services. Surgery of the War* (London: His Majesty's Stationery Office, 1922), 2–5.

30. Macpherson, *History of the Great War*, I, 101.

31. Macpherson, *History of the Great War*, I, 42.

32. Melville, "Casualties in Modern War," 358. For similar information, see Gaston Bodart, *Militar-historisches kriegs-lexikon (1618–1905)* (Liepzig: C. W. Stern, 1908).

33. Macpherson, "The Removal of Sick and Wounded," 89–90; Maurice, *System of Field Manoeuvers*, 15.

34. Melville, "Casualties in Modern War," 359.

35. Macpherson, "Removal of Sick and Wounded," 93–94; Straub, *Medical Service in Campaign*, 54–56.

36. Ford, "Notes on Organization and Equipment," 675.

37. Gore, "The Ambulance in War," 357; Colin, *The Transformations of War*, 322–55.

38. Quoted in Gore, "The Ambulance in War," 356; Havard, "Litter and Ambulance Transportation," 45.

39. Quoted in Gore, "The Ambulance in War," 356.

40. Quoted in Gore, "The Ambulance in War," 356.

41. Quoted in Bird, *Errand of Mercy*, 304–5, 306.

42. Macpherson, "The Removal of Sick and Wounded," 87.

43. Jones, "Report upon the Transport of Sick and Wounded," 589.

44. Melville, "Casualties in Modern War," 360; Macpherson, "Removal of Sick and Wounded," 87.

45. Ford, "Notes on Organization and Equipment," 672.

46. Kimball, "Transportation of the Wounded in War," 194.

47. Gore, "The Ambulance in War," 353; Ford, "Notes on Organization and Equipment," 670.

48. Ford, "Notes on Organization and Equipment," 682–84.

49. [Anonymous], "Ambulance Dogs," *British Medical Journal*, II (1904), 1589–90; [Anonymous], "Ambulance Dogs," *British Medical Journal*, I (1917), 16; E. C. Jones, "Military Dogs," *Military Surgeon*, XL (1917), 395–400.

50. Clyde Sinclair Ford, "The Military Motor Ambulance," *Proceedings*, Association of Military Surgeons of the United States, XII (1903), 72.

51. Katherine T. Barkley, *The Ambulance: The Story of Emergency Transportation of Sick and Wounded Through the Centuries* (Hicksville, New York: Exposition Press, 1978), 102–3; Norman Miller Cary, Jr., *The Use of the Motor Vehicle in the United States Army, 1899–1939* (Athens, Georgia: Unpublished Ph.D. Dissertation, University of Georgia, 1980), 6–7.

52. United States Government, War Department, "Report of the Secretary of War for the Year 1895," *Annual Reports of the War Department for the Fiscal Year Ended June 30, 1895* (Washington, D.C.: Government Printing Office, 1895), I, 69.

53. Cary, *Use of the Motor Vehicle*, 13.

54. Ford, "Military Motor Ambulance," 75–79.

55. Ford, "Military Motor Ambulance," 76.

56. Ford, "Military Motor Ambulance," 75.

57. James A. Tobey, *The Medical Department of the Army: Its History, Activities and Organization* (Baltimore: Johns Hopkins University Press, 1927), 33–34.

58. Percy M. Ashburn, *A History of the Medical Department of the United States Army* (Boston: Houghton Mifflin, 1929), 233–34; United States Government, War Department, "Report of the Quartermaster General," *Annual Reports of the War Department for the Fiscal Year Ended June 30, 1917* (Washington, D.C.: Government Printing Office, 1917), 74; Cary, *Use of the Motor Vehicle*, 101–103.

59. Ford, "Notes on Organization and Equipment," 686–87.

60. Cary, *Use of the Motor Vehicle*, 89–95.

5. NEW CHALLENGES

1. Russell F. Weigley, *The American Way of War: A History of United States Military Strategy and Policy* (New York: Macmillan, 1973), 200.

2. William Mitchell, *Memories of World War I: "From Start to Finish of Our Greatest War"* (New York: Random House, 1960), 10.

3. Archibald Magill Fauntleroy, *Report on the Medico-Military Aspects of the European War: From Observations Taken Behind the Allied Armies in France* (Washington, D.C.: Government Printing Office, 1915), 118.

4. Eric J. Leed, *No Man's Land: Combat and Identity in World War I* (Cambridge: Cambridge University Press, 1979), 8, 20, 98–100.

5. Martin Middlebrook, *The First Day on the Somme, 1 July 1916* (New York: Norton, 1972), 45–47; J. S. Smith, *Trench Warfare: A Manual for Officers and Men* (New York: Dutton, 1917), 1–24, 45–48, 56–67; Arthur Graham Butler, *The Australian Army Medical Services in the War of 1914–1918* (3 vols.; Canberra: Australian War Memorial, 1940), II, 35.

6. T. J. Mitchell, "Some Guiding Principles in the Evacuation of Casualties," *Journal of the Royal Army Medical Corps*, XLVII (1926), 29; James A. Tobey, *The Medical Department of the Army: Its History, Activities and Organization* (Baltimore: Johns Hopkins University Press, 1927), 41–42.

7. Frank T. Woodbury, "The Ambulance Company," *Military Surgeon*, XXXIV (1914), 529.

8. General Surgeon Dr. Bulius, "The Medical Service of the Third Army in the Battle of the Marne (September 6–10, 1914)," *Military Surgeon*, LV (1924), 553–67; Middlebrook, *First Day on the Somme*, 191, 251; Butler, *Australian Army Medical Services*, II, 135.

9. Butler, *Australian Army Medical Services*, II, 64.

10. Anderson Robert Dillon Carbery, *The New Zealand Medical Service in the Great War, 1914–1918* (Auckland: Whitcombe and Tombs, 1924), 55–56, 65–66.

11. Middlebrook, *First Day on the Somme*, 253–54, 267.

12. Joseph A. Blake, "Early Experience in the War," *Military Surgeon*, XLV (1919), 629–30; Arthur F. Hurst, *Medical Diseases of the War* (London: Edward Arnold, 1918), 250–80.

13. Percy L. Jones, "The Evacuation of Wounded by Motor Vehicles in the Rear Section of the Advance Zone," *War Medicine*, Paris, II (1918), 199–200; [Anonymous], "The Ambulance Services of the Warring Nations," *American Medicine*, XXI (1915), 776; John Gilmour, "Transportation of Wounded," *Military Surgeon*, XLII (1918), 12.

14. Woodbury, "The Ambulance Company," 516.

15. Woodbury, "The Ambulance Company," 516.

16. Denis Winter, *Death's Men: Soldiers of the Great War* (London: Allen Lane, 1978), 197.

17. [Doc.], "The Evolution of Stretcher-Bearing in This War," *University of Durham College of Medicine Gazette*, XVII (1917), 39–40; Carbery, *New Zealand Medical Service*, 46.

18. George de Tarnowsky, *Military Surgery of the Zone of the Advance* (Philadelphia: Lea and Febiger, 1918), 47.

19. de Tarnowsky, *Military Surgery*, 42; M. W. Ireland (ed.), *The Medical Department of the United States Army in the World War, 1917–1918*, vol. VIII, *Field Operations* (Washington, D.C.: Government Printing Office, 1925), 111–49.

20. de Tarnowsky, *Military Surgery*, 30–41.

21. Gilmour, "Transportation of Wounded," 3; James A. Moss, *Trench Warfare* (Menasha, Wisconsin: George Banta, 1917), 29.

22. Percy M. Ashburn, *A History of the Medical Department of the United States Army* (Boston: Houghton Mifflin, 1929), 347; Edmund L. Gross, "The Transportation of the Wounded," *Boston Medical and Surgical Journal*, CLXXIII (1915), 1–3; William G. Macpherson, *History of the Great War Based on Official Documents*, vol. II, *Medical Services, General History* (London: His Majesty's Stationery Office, 1923), 16–22.

23. Gross, "Transportation of the Wounded," 1–3; John H. Plumridge, *Hospital Ships and Ambulance Trains* (London: Seeley, Service, 1975), 114–17; Butler, *Australian Army Medical Services*, II, 272–93; Macpherson, *History of the Great War*, II, 568–74.

24. Macpherson, *History of the Great War*, IV, 647–53.

25. Gilmour, "Transportation of Wounded," 7–8; Carbery, *New Zealand Medical Service*, 46.

26. Butler, *Australian Army Medical Services*, II, 312.

27. Butler, *Australian Army Medical Services*, II, 13–14; Eloise Engle, *Medic: America's Medical Soldiers, Sailors and Airmen in Peace and War* (New York: John Day, 1967), 39; J. A. Nydegger, "Some Recent Medical Observations in the European War Zone," *Medical Record*, XC (1916), 318–19; A. E. Shipley, *The Minor Horrors of War* (3d ed.; London: Smith, Elder, 1916), 1–35, 132–42; Edward B. Vedder, *Sanitation for Medical Officers* (Philadelphia: Lea and Febiger, 1917), 105–29.

28. Butler, *Australian Army Medical Services*, II, 312.

29. H. Bayon, "Notes from the South African Hospital at Cannes, France: The Removal of Wounded from the Battlefield to Base Hospital," *South African Medical Journal*, XIII (1915), 254.

30. [Doc.], "Evolution of Stretcher-Bearing in This War," 35–36; Middlebrook, *First Day on the Somme*, 230–32.

31. E. K. Johnstone, "From 'Over the Top' to the 'C.C.S.,'" *Military Surgeon*, XLI (1917), 698; Robert B. Osgood, "The Transport Splints of the American Expeditionary Forces," *Military Surgeon*, XLV (1919), 588–600.

32. Gross, "Transportation of the Wounded," 4.

33. Gross, "Transportation of the Wounded," 4.

34. Winter, *Death's Men*, 197.

35. H. E. R. James and C. E. Pollock, "The Clearing Hospital and the Evacuation of Sick and Wounded from an Army in the Field," *Journal of the Royal Army Medical Corps*, XVIII (1912), 55–57; [Anonymous], "The War: Its Hospital, Medical and Nursing Aspects," *Modern Hospital*, IX (1917), 443–44; [Anonymous], "What Is Done for the Wounded: How They Are Collected at the Front and Transferred to the Permanent Hospitals," *Scientific American*, LXXXI (1916), 196; Macpherson, *History of the Great War*, I, 208–47; II, 42–51, 349.

36. H. Rouvillois, "The H.O.E. in the French Army (Primary and Secondary) Evacuation Hospitals," *Military Surgeon*, LVI (1925), 531.

37. Douglas A. Rund and Tondra S. Rausch, *Triage* (St. Louis: Mosby, 1981),

3–4; *Oxford English Dictionary* (Oxford: Clarendon Press, 1933), XI, 334; *Emergency War Medicine* (Washington, D.C.: Government Printing Office, 1975), 156.

38. *Emergency War Medicine*, 533–35.

39. Ireland, *Medical Department*, III, 143.

40. J. H. Ford, "First-Aid and Dressing Stations in Battle in the Austro-Hungarian Army," *Military Surgeon*, XLI (1917), 181.

41. Ford, "First-Aid and Dressing Stations in Battle," 181–82.

42. Ford, "First-Aid and Dressing Stations in Battle," 183–85.

43. Otto Von Schjerning, "The Activities and Achievements of Medical Officers of the German Army During the War: Introduction to the 'Handbook of Medical Experiences in the World War,'" *Military Surgeon*, XLVI (1920), 432.

44. General Surgeon Dr. Altgelt, "The Preparation for the Great German Offensive on the Western Front in the Spring of 1918," *Military Surgeon*, LIV (1924), 600–601, 606.

45. Fielding H. Garrison, "The German Medical History of the War," *Military Surgeon*, XLVI (1920), 428.

46. Ludwig Fritz Haber, *The Poisonous Cloud: Chemical Warfare in the First World War* (New York: Oxford University Press, 1986), 18–19; H. L. Gilchrist, *A Comparative Study of Warfare Gases: Their History, Description and Medical Aspects* (Washington, D.C.: Government Printing Office, 1925), 2.

47. Cyril B. Falls, *The First World War* (London: Longmans, Green, 1960), 91–93; Alistair Horne, *The Price of Glory: Verdun 1916* (London: Macmillan, 1962), 284; Ludwig Fritz Haber, *The Chemical Industry, 1900–1930* (Oxford: Clarendon Press, 1971), 208–9; Amos A. Fries and Clarence J. West, *Chemical Warfare* (New York: McGraw Hill, 1921), 16–17; Victor Lefebure, *The Riddle of the Rhine: Chemical Strategy in Peace and War* (New York: Dutton, 1923), 39–40; Moss, *Trench Warfare*, 155; Macpherson, *History of the Great War*, II, 395–423.

48. Haber, *Poisonous Cloud*, 239–43; H. L. Gilchrist, *A Comparative Study of World War Casualties from Gas and Other Weapons* (Washington, D.C.: Government Printing Office, 1928), 6; Augustin M. Prentiss, *Chemicals in War: A Treatise on Chemical Warfare* (New York: McGraw-Hill, 1937), 653–55; Lefebure, *Riddle of the Rhine*, 48–65.

49. Joseph Catton, "Gas Warfare—Its Aftermath," *Military Surgeon*, XLV (1919), 65; H. L. Gilchrist, "Chemical Warfare and Its Medical Significance," *Military Surgeon*, XLIII (1928), 477–92; Haber, *Poisonous Cloud*, 57, 239; Prentiss, *Chemicals in War*, 653–55.

50. Fries and West, *Chemical Warfare*, 195–236; Van H. Manning, *War Gas Investigations* (Washington, D.C.: Government Printing Office, 1919), 11–13, 18–21; M. Abbott, "Gas in War," *Medical Press*, CVII (1919), 221–23, 238–41.

51. Quoted in Winter, *Death's Men*, 123.

52. J. A. Nydegger, "Some Recent Medical Observations," 319; Edward B. Vedder, *The Medical Aspects of Chemical Warfare* (Baltimore: Williams and Wilkins, 1925), 77–123; M. C. Winternitz, *Collected Studies on the Pathology of War Gas Poisoning* (New Haven, Connecticut: Yale University Press, 1920), 33–66; Great Britain, Medical Research Committee, *An Atlas of Gas Poisoning* (Great Britain: American Red Cross, 1918).

53. Edward S. Farrow, *Gas Warfare* (New York: Dutton, 1920), 222–24.

54. Alfred de Roulet, "Organization of Divisional Medical Service for Handling Gas Casualties," *Military Surgeon*, LVIII (1926), 160–61; Vedder, *Medical Aspects of Chemical Warfare*, 125–66; Winternitz, *Collected Studies*, 99–114.

55. Fries and West, *Chemical Warfare*, 419–22; Vedder, *Medical Aspects of Chemical Warfare*, 5; H. L. Gilchrist, *Report on the After Effects of Warfare Gases* (Washington, D.C.: Chemical Warfare Service, 1923), 36–88.

56. Farrow, *Gas Warfare*, 225–26.

57. Haber, *Poisonous Cloud*, 239–58; Vedder, *Medical Aspects of Chemical Warfare*, 239–43; Gilchrist, *Comparative Study of Warfare Gases*, 88–95; Ireland, *Medical Department*, III, 146–47.

6. TRIALS OF EVACUATION

1. H. Bayon, "Notes from the South African Hospital at Cannes, France: The Removal of Wounded from the Battlefield to Base Hospital," *South African Medical Journal*, XIII (1915), 252.

2. Bayon, "Notes from the South African Hospital at Cannes," 252; F. W. Foxworthy, "Progress in War Transportation: The Motor Ambulance, the Motor Hospital and Motor Surgery," *Progress in War Transportation*, XXXV (1914), 420; R. H. Beadon, *The Royal Army Service Corps: A History of Transport and Supply in the British Army* (2 vols.; Cambridge: Cambridge University Press, 1931), II, 90.

3. Arthur Graham Butler, *The Australian Army Medical Services in the War of 1914–1918* (3 vols.; Canberra; Australian War Memorial, 1940), II, 288.

4. Bayon, "Notes from the South African Hospital at Cannes," 252.

5. T. J. Mitchell, "Some Guiding Principles in the Evacuation of Casualties," *Journal of the Royal Army Medical Corps*, XLVII (1926), 27.

6. H. Masswac Buist, "Ambulance Work at the Front," *British Medical Journal*, II (1914), 642; W. C. Beevor, "The Removal of Sick and Wounded in Motor-Lorries: A Warning and Counter Proposal," *Journal of the Royal Army Medical Corps*, XXIII (1914), 66–68.

7. Buist, "Ambulance Work at the Front," 642; H. Masswac Buist, "Motor Ambulances in War Service," *British Medical Journal*, II (1914), 546.

8. Beevor, "Removal of Sick and Wounded in Motor-Lorries," 66–68.

9. Anderson Robert Dillon Carbery, *The New Zealand Medical Service in the Great War, 1914–1918* (Auckland: Whitcombe and Tombs, 1924), 23.

10. Foxworthy, "Progress in War Transportation," 421, 425.

11. Layton John Blenkinsop and J. W. Rainey (eds.), *History of the Great War Based on Official Documents. Veterinary Services* (London: His Majesty's Stationery Office, 1925), 70, 508, 515.

12. Buist, "Ambulance Work at the Front," 642; William G. Macpherson, *History of the Great War Based on Official Documents*, vol. IV, *Medical Services. General History* (London: His Majesty's Stationery Office, 1924), 608–11.

13. G. Gree, "A Single Divisional Field Ambulance," *Journal of the Royal Army Medical Corps*, XXIII (1914), 223; Foxworthy, "Progress in War Transportation," 420.

14. G. Poe, "The Transportation of Wounded Men from the Point of View of Motor Ambulance Convoys," *War Medicine*, II (1918), 191–93.

15. Katherine T. Barkley, *The Ambulance: The Story of Emergency Transportation of Sick and Wounded Through the Centuries* (Hicksville, New York: Exposition Press, 1978), 103–4.

16. Buist, "Motor Ambulances in War Service," 545.

17. Edmund L. Gross, "The Transportation of the Wounded," *Boston Medical and Surgical Journal*, CLXXIII (1915), 6.

18. H. Masswac Buist, "Motor Ambulances for War Service," *British Medical Journal*, I (1915), 42–43.

19. Stephen Thorn, "Notes, Experiences and Suggestions on the Automobile Ambulance Service of a Modern Army in the Field," *Military Surgeon*, XLI (1917), 415; American Ambulance Field Service, *Friends of France: The Field Service of the American Ambulance Described by Its Members* (Boston: Houghton Mifflin, 1916), 149.

20. American Ambulance Field Service, *Friends of France*, 373; Guy Emerson Bowerman, Jr., *The Compensations of War: The Diary of an Ambulance Driver During the Great War* (Austin: University of Texas Press, 1983), 16; M. W. Ireland (ed.), *The Medical Department of the United States Army in the World War*, vol. VIII, *Field Operations* (Washington, D.C.: Government Printing Office, 1925), 119–20.

21. Quoted in A. Piatt Andrew, "The Genesis of the American Ambulance Service with the French Army, 1915–1917," *Military Surgeon*, LVII (1925), 375.

22. Gross, "Transportation of the Wounded," 4–7.

23. Quoted in Jay W. Grissinger, "Field Service," *Military Surgeon*, LXI (1927), 461–62.

24. Thorn, "Notes, Experiences and Suggestions," 417, 420.

25. Thorn, "Notes, Experiences and Suggestions," 418.

26. Thorn, "Notes, Experiences and Suggestions," 419.

27. Andrew, "Genesis of the American Ambulance Service," 363–64; James R. Judd, *With the American Ambulance in France* (Honolulu: Star-Bulletin Press, 1919).

28. Andrew, "Genesis of the American Ambulance Service," 366–67.

29. American Ambulance Field Service, *Friends of France*, 1–4; Ireland, *Medical Department*, VIII, 223–24.

30. Bowerman, *Compensations of War*, 115–16, 119.

31. Bowerman, *Compensations of War*, chapter 15; Malcolm Cowley, *Exile's Return* (New York: Viking, 1972).

32. Julien H. Bryan, *Ambulance 464: Encore des Blessés* (New York: Macmillan, 1918), viii; William M. L. Coplin, *American Red Cross Base Hospital No. 38, Organized Under the Auspices of the Jefferson Medical College and Hospital, Stationed at Nantes, France, 1918–1919* (Philadelphia: E. A. Wright, 1923); Henry James, *Within the Rim, and Other Essays, 1914–1915* (London: W. Collins, 1918).

33. Edwin Wilson Morse, *The Vanguard of American Volunteers in the Fighting Lines and in Humanitarian Service, August, 1914–April, 1917* (New York: Scribner, 1918), 160; Bowerman, *Compensations of War*, 7.

34. American Ambulance Field Service, *Friends of France*, 41.

35. Thorn, "Notes, Experiences and Suggestions," 420–21; Philip Dana Orcutt, *The White Road of Mystery: The Note-book of an American Ambulancier* (New York: John Lane, 1918), 47–48.

36. Thorn, "Notes, Experiences and Suggestions," 423; Ireland, *Medical Department*, VIII, 229–30; A Member of the Unit, *The Story of United States Army Base Hospital No. 5* (Cambridge: Cambridge University Press, 1919), 2–3.

37. Buist, "Motor Ambulances for War Service," 42–43; Mitchell, "Some Guiding Principles in the Evacuation of Casualties," 26; Macpherson, *History of the Great War*, IV, 625.

38. Andrew, "Genesis of the American Ambulance Service," 371–72.

39. Andrew, "Genesis of the American Ambulance Service," 372–73.

40. Andrew, "Genesis of the American Ambulance Service," 376–77; Ireland, *Medical Department*, VIII, 34, 211, 231.

41. Ireland, *Medical Department*, VIII, 119.

42. Francis A. Winter, "The American Red Cross with the A.E.F.," *Military Surgeon*, XLIV (1919), 549–50; Ireland, *Medical Department*, VIII, 33, 36.

43. Sanford H. Wadhams and Arnold D. Tuttle, "Some of the Early Problems of the Medical Department," *Military Surgeon*, XLV (1919), 636.

44. Fielding H. Garrison, "Notes on the History of Military Medicine," *Military Surgeon*, LI (1922), 210; Wadhams and Tuttle, "Some Early Problems of the Medical Department," 636.

45. J. R. Kean, "Evacuation of the American Wounded in the Aisne-Marne Battles, June and July, 1918," *Military Surgeon*, LVI (1925), 488.

46. Wadhams and Tuttle, "Some Early Problems of the Medical Department," 657–58; Ireland, *Medical Department*, VIII, 31; Carter Henry Harrison, *With the American Red Cross in France, 1918–1919* (Chicago: Ralph Fletcher Seymour, 1947), 54–55; Charles H. Kaletzki (ed.), *Official History: U.S.A. Base Hospital No. 31 of Youngstown, Ohio, and Hospital Unit "G" of Syracuse University* (Syracuse, New York: Craftsmen Press, 1919).

47. Wadhams and Tuttle, "Some Early Problems of the Medical Department," 658–60.

48. [Editor], "Comment," *Military Surgeon*, XLIV (1919), 256–57.

49. Percy M. Ashburn, *A History of the Medical Department of the United States Army* (Boston: Houghton Mifflin, 1929), 342.

50. George Cheever Shattuck, "Medical Work in the British Armies in France," *Military Surgeon*, XLV (1919), 251–52.

51. J. A. Murphy, "Naval Transportation of Army Sick and Wounded Overseas," *Military Surgeon*, XLIV (1919), 178–82.

52. Martin L. Van Creveld, *Supplying War: Logistics from Wallenstein to Patton* (Cambridge: Cambridge University Press, 1977), 109–41.

53. George A. Moore, *The Birth and Early Days of Our Ambulance Trains in France, August, 1914, to April, 1915* (London: John Bale Sons and Danielsson, 1922), 4; John Gilmour, "Transportation of Wounded," *Military Surgeon*, XLII (1918), 11–12.

54. Gross, "Transportation of the Wounded," 6.

55. Gross, "Transportation of the Wounded," 7; Bayon, "Notes from the vol. XI, *Surgery* (Washington, D.C.: Government Printing Office, 1927), 50; South African Hospital at Cannes," 252.

56. Moore, *Birth and Early Days of Our Ambulance Trains*, 6–8, 16.

57. Moore, *Birth and Early Days of Our Ambulance Trains*, 18.

58. Moore, *Birth and Early Days of Our Ambulance Trains*, 19.

59. R. W. D. Leslie, "Improvised Ambulance Trains," *Journal of the Royal Army Medical Corps*, XXXIV (1920), 431–34; F. L. Pleadwell, "British Ambulance Trains," *Military Surgeon*, XLVI (1920), 57.

60. Howard Clarke, "American Hospital Trains in France," *Medical Times*, XLVI (1918), 117.

61. Ashburn, *History of the Medical Department*, 343.

62. Clarke, "American Hospital Trains in France," 117; Pleadwell, "British Ambulance Trains," 51-58.

63. Caswell A. Mayo, "Army Hospital Trains," *New York Medical Journal*, CIX (1919), 594–97.

7. Lessons Learned

1. M. W. Ireland (ed.), *The Medical Department of the United States Army in the World War, 1917–1918*, vol. XI, *Surgery* (Washington, D.C.: Government Printing Office, 1927), 50; Lieutenant Colonel Garbowski, "Evacuation in a War of Movement," *Journal of the Royal Army Medical Corps*, XLIX (1927), 338; Albert G. Love, "A Brief Summary of the Vital Statistics of the U.S. Army During the World War," *Military Surgeon*, XLVII (1920), 244–60.

2. William S. Bainbridge, "Some Lessons of the World War in Medicine and Surgery from the German Viewpoint," *Military Surgeon*, XLIX (1921), 366–67; Harold Dearden, *Medicine and Duty: A War Diary* (London: Heinemann, 1928), 13; Bruce D. Ragsdale, "Gunshot Wounds: A Historical Perspective," *Military Medicine*, CXLIX (1984), 310.

3. James C. Beyer (ed.), *Wound Ballistics* (Washington, D.C.: Department of the Army, 1962), 145; William G. Macpherson, *History of the Great War Based on Official Documents*, vol. I, *Medical Services. Surgery of the War* (London: His Majesty's Stationery Office, 1922), 20–26; Ireland, *Medical Department*, XI, 45–54.

4. L. B. Wilson, "Dispersion of Bullet Energy in Relation to Wound Effects," *Military Surgeon*, XLIX (1921), 241–51; Archibald Magill Fauntleroy, *Report on the Medico-Military Aspects of the European War: From Observations Taken Behind the Allied Armies in France* (Washington, D.C.: Government Printing Office, 1915), 10–12.

5. Ireland, *Medical Department*, XI, xxxii.

6. Bainbridge, "Some Lessons of the World War in Medicine and Surgery," 371; Fielding H. Garrison, "Notes on the History of Military Medicine," *Military Surgeon*, LI (1922), 212; Marie Louis Fermin Duguet, "General Organization of the Treatment and Evacuation of Wounded with Fractures, in the Area of the Front," *Military Surgeon*, LIII (1923), 574; Owen H. Wangensteen, Sarah D.

Wangensteen, and Charles F. Klinger, "Wound Management of Ambrose Paré and Dominique Larrey, Great French Military Surgeons of the 16th and 19th Centuries," *Bulletin of the History of Medicine*, XLVI (1972), 207–34.

7. Garbowski, "Evacuation in a War of Movement," 339–40.

8. George de Tarnowsky, "Advance Surgical Formations — Modifications Which Seem Necessary in the Light of the German Offensive of March–July, 1918," *Military Surgeon*, XLIV (1919), 245–48; Ireland, *Medical Department*, VIII, 32–33.

9. de Tarnowsky, "Advance Surgical Formations," 245–48.

10. de Tarnowsky, "Advance Surgical Formations," 249–55.

11. [Editor], "Comment," *Military Surgeon*, XLIV (1919), 256–57.

12. Bailey K. Ashford, "A Lecture on Field Hospitals," *Military Surgeon*, XLIV (1919), 560–61; Hans Zinsser, "The Medical Corps in Peace and War," *Military Surgeon*, LXIII (1928), 153–66.

13. T. L. Rhoads, "Principles of Evacuation," *Military Surgeon*, LIV (1924), 299–300.

14. H. Rouvillois, "The H.O.E. in the French Army (Primary and Secondary) Evacuation Hospitals," *Military Surgeon*, LVI (1925), 529–57; Elliott C. Cutler, "The Organization, Function and Operation of an Evacuation Hospital," *Military Surgeon*, XLVI (1920), 9–32.

15. Edward L. Munson, *The Principles of Sanitary Tactics: A Handbook on the Use of Medical Department Detachments and Organizations in Campaign* (Menasha, Wisconsin: George Banta, 1917), 59–60; Garbowski, "Evacuation in a War of Movement," 353–54.

16. John F. Morrison and Edward L. Munson, *A Study in Troop Leading and Management of the Sanitary Service in War* (Menasha, Wisconsin: George Banta, 1918).

17. Rhoads, "Principles of Evacuation," 343.

18. Fred H. Bloomhardt, "Transportation for Medical Department in Campaign in the Philippine Islands," *Military Surgeon*, LVI (1925), 169–71.

19. H. L. Gilchrist, *Chemical Warfare: Medical Aspects; Their History; Classifications; Symptoms Produced; Pathology and Treatment* (Washington, D.C.: Government Printing Office, 1922); L. F. Haber, *The Poisonous Cloud: Chemical Warfare in the First World War* (New York: Oxford University Press, 1986); Norman Fenton, *Shell Shock and Its Aftermath* (St. Louis: C. V. Mosby, 1926); E. E. Southard, *Shell-Shock and Other Neuropsychiatric Problems in 589 Case Histories from the War Literature, 1914–1918* (Boston: W. M. Leonard, 1919); Alexis Carrel and G. Dehelly, *The Treatment of Infected Wounds* (New York: P. B. Hoeber, 1917); J. W. Kerr, "Some Influences of the World War on the Future of National Health," *Military Surgeon*, XLIV (1921), 125–32; J. Smyth, "Lessons of the War May Be Applicable to Civil Practice," *Military Surgeon*, XLVII (1920), 100–108; Ireland, *Medical Department*, XI, 185–211.

20. Ashford, "Lecture on Field Hospitals," 558–60.

21. Harry George Armstrong, *Principles and Practice of Aviation Medicine* (3d ed.; Baltimore: Williams and Wilkins, 1952); David M. Lam, "To Pop a Balloon: Aeromedical Evacuation in the 1870 Siege of Paris," *Aviation, Space, and Environ-*

mental Medicine, LIX (1988), 988–91; Fritz Bauer, "Experiments with Aeroplanes Used by the Medical Services in War and in Peace Time," *Journal of the Royal Army Medical Corps*, LII (1929), 81–82; E. M. Cowell, "Air Ambulances," *Journal of the Royal Army Medical Corps*, LXII (1934), 260–61; Robert F. Futrell, *Development of Aeromedical Evacuation in the U.S.A.F., 1909–1960* (United States Air Force Historical Division: Research Studies Institute Air University, 1960), 5–6.

22. Futrell, *Development of Aeromedical Evacuation*, 4–6.

23. Bauer, "Experiments With Aeroplanes," 82.

24. Cowell, "Air Ambulances," 261–62; Bauer, "Experiments with Aeroplanes," 84.

25. Bauer, "Experiments with Aeroplanes," 83; [Anonymous], "Military Medical Aeroplanes," *British Medical Journal*, II (1919), 785–86.

26. Eran Dolev, "First Recorded Aeromedical Evacuation in the British Army — The True Story," *Journal of the Royal Army Medical Corps*, CXXXII (1986), 34–36.

27. J. C. Burns, "A Note on the Evacuation of Service Casualties by Air," *Journal of the Royal Army Medical Corps*, XLVI (1926), 202–5.

28. F. R. Guilford and B. J. Soboroff, "Air Evacuation: An Historical Review," *Journal of Aviation Medicine*, XVIII (1947), 601–16; Munro, "Use of the Aeroplane in the Medical Services," 7–9; Bauer, "Experiments with Aeroplanes," 84; T. E. Darby, "Aeroplane Ambulance Evacuation," *Military Surgeon*, LXXI (1932), 163.

29. Munro, "Use of the Aeroplane in the Medical Services," 11–12; Cowell, "Air Ambulances," 260.

30. Bauer, "Experiments with Aeroplanes," 85.

31. Norvelle Wallace Sharpe, "The Ambulance Airship," *Annals of Surgery*, LXVIII (1918), 526–27.

32. Munro, "Use of the Aeroplane in the Medical Services," 11.

33. S. M. Strong, "Aero Ambulance," *Military Surgeon*, LXIV (1919), 361–62.

34. Futrell, *Development of Aeromedical Evacuation*, 12–15.

35. L. H. Bauer, "The Development of Commercial Aeronautics and of the Airplane Ambulance," *Military Surgeon*, LXVI (1930), 170–73.

36. Darby, "Aeroplane Ambulance Evacuation," 163–64; M. W. Ireland, "The Medical Service in a Theatre of Operations," *Military Surgeon*, LXII (1928), 585; C. L. Beaven, "New Ambulance Airplane for U.S. Army Air Corps," *Military Surgeon*, LXVIII (1931), 777–80.

37. Darby, "Aeroplane Ambulance Evacuation," 164.

38. Darby, "Aeroplane Ambulance Evacuation," 165–66; Robert K. Simpson, "The Airplane Ambulance — Its Use in War," *Military Surgeon*, LXIV (1929), 35–48.

39. Darby, "Aeroplane Ambulance Evacuation," 167–68.

40. Darby, "Aeroplane Ambulance Evacuation," 169.

Selected Bibliography

This book has been researched chiefly from books, pamphlets, and journal articles of the nineteenth and early twentieth centuries. To assist the interested reader, I have included complete listings of books and pamphlets used, as well as of certain general works that afford insight into the period and the subject as a whole, and I have listed all journals cited in the text and notes.

JOURNALS CITED IN TEXT AND NOTES

Albany Medical Annals
American Cyclopedia of Practical Medicine and Surgery
American Medicine
Annals of Emergency Medicine
Annals of Medical History
Annals of Surgery
Army Ordnance
Automobile
Automotor and Horseless Vehicle Journal
Aviation, Space, and Environmental Medicine
Boston Medical and Surgical Journal
British Medical Journal
Brooklyn Medical Journal
Bulletin, New York Academy of Medicine
Bulletin of the History of Medicine
Caduceus
Cavalry Journal
Chicago Medical Journal and Examiner
Ciba Symposia
Civil War Times
Cleveland Medical Journal
Commercial Vehicle
Cooper's Vehicle Journal
Cycle and Automobile Trade Journal

Edinburgh Medical Journal
Engineering News
Indian Journal of Medicine and the Physical Sciences
Indian Medical Gazette, Calcutta
Infantry Journal
Injury
International Congress of Charities, Corrections and Philanthropy
Journal of the American Medical Association
Journal of Aviation Medicine
Journal of Emergency Medicine
Journal of the History of Medicine
Journal of Military History
Journal of the Oklahoma State Medical Association
Journal of the Royal Army Medical Corps
Journal of the Royal College of Surgeons of Edinburgh
Journal of the Royal United Service Institution
Lancet
Medical Heritage
Medical History
Medical Press
Medical Record
Medical Review
Medical Times
Military Affairs
Military Collector and Historian
Military Medicine
Military Surgeon
Modern Hospital
New Orleans Medical and Surgical Journal
New York Medical Journal
New York State Journal of Medicine
New Zealand Medical Journal
North American Review
Philadelphia Medical Journal
Proceedings, Association of Military Surgeons of the United States
Proceedings, International Congress of the History of Medicine
Progress in War Transportation
Quartermaster Review
Railway Surgeon
Report, Army Medical Department, London
Sanitarian
Scientific American
South African Medical Journal
Transactions, Indian Medical Congress
Transactions, International Medical Congress
Transactions, Medical Society of the State of New York
Transactions, National Association for the Promotion of Social Science
United States National Museum Bulletin

University of Durham College of Medicine Gazette
Virginia Medical Monthly
War Medicine
Wood's Medical and Surgical Monographs

BOOKS AND PAMPHLETS

Abrahamson, James L. *American Arms for a New Century: Making of a Great Military Power*. New York: Free Press, 1981.

Adams, George W. *Doctors in Blue: The Medical History of the Union Army in the Civil War*. New York: Henry Schuman, 1952.

Allcott, Louisa M. *Hospital Sketches*. Boston: James Redpath, 1863.

Allen, Paul. *History of the Expedition Under the Command of Captains Lewis and Clark, to the Sources of the Missouri, Thence Across the Rocky Mountains and Down the River Columbia to the Pacific Ocean. Performed During the Years 1804–5–6, by Order of the Government of the United States*. Philadelphia: Bradford and Inskeep, 1817.

Ambrose, Stephen E. *Upton and the Army*. Baton Rouge: Louisiana State University Press, 1964.

American Ambulance Field Service. *Diary of Section VIII: American Ambulance Field Service*. Boston: T. Todd, 1917.

American Ambulance Field Service. *Friends of France: The Field Service of the American Ambulance Described by Its Members*. Boston: Houghton Mifflin, 1916.

American Ambulance Field Service. *History of the American Field Service in France: "Friends of France," 1914–1917*. 3 vols.; Boston: Houghton Mifflin, 1920.

Appia, P. L. *The Ambulance Surgeon or Practical Observations on Gunshot Wounds*. Edinburgh: Adams and Charles Black, 1862.

Armstrong, Harry George. *Principles and Practice of Aviation Medicine*. 3d ed.; Baltimore: Williams and Wilkins, 1952.

Ashburn, Percy M. *A History of the Medical Department of the United States Army*. Boston: Houghton Mifflin, 1929.

Ashworth, Tony. *Trench Warfare 1914–1918: The Live and Let Live System*. New York: Holmes and Meier, 1980.

Ayres, Leonard P. *The War with Germany: A Statistical Survey*. Washington, D.C.: Government Printing Office, 1919.

Baker, Colonel Chauncey B. *Motor Transportation for the Army*. Washington, D.C.: Government Printing Office, 1917.

Ballentine, George. *The Mexican War, by an English Soldier. Comprising Incidents of the Adventures in the United States and Mexico with the American Army*. New York: W. A. Townsend, 1853.

Ballingall, George. *Outlines of Military Surgery*. Edinburgh: Adam and Charles Black, 1855.

Barkley, Katherine T. *The Ambulance: The Story of Emergency Transportation of Sick and Wounded Through the Centuries*. Hicksville, New York: Exposition Press, 1978.

Barringer, Emily D. *Bowery to Bellevue: The Story of New York's First Woman Ambulance Surgeon*. New York: Norton, 1950.

Bartlett, John R. *Personal Narrative of Explorations and Incidents in Texas.* 2 vols.; New York: Rio Grande Press, 1854.

Barton, Clara. *The Red Cross: A History of This Remarkable Movement in the Interest of Humanity.* Washington, D.C.: American National Red Cross, 1898.

Barton, Clara. *The Red Cross in Peace and War.* Meriden, Connecticut: Journal Publishing, 1912.

Barton, William E. *The Life of Clara Barton, Founder of the American Red Cross.* 2 vols.; New York: AMS Press, 1969.

Baudens, Lucien. *On Military and Camp Hospitals and the Health of Troops in the Field: Being the Results of a Commission To Inspect the Sanitary Arrangements of the French Army and Incidentally of Other Armies in the Crimean War.* New York: Bailliere, 1862.

Baum, Charles. *Les trains sanitaires en Russie et en Autriche-Hongrie.* Paris: n.p., 1879.

Baxter, J. H. (comp.). *Statistics, Medical and Anthropological of the Provost-Marshal-General's Bureau.* Washington, D.C.: Government Printing Office, 1875.

Baylen, Joseph O., and Alan Conway (eds.). *Soldier-Surgeon. The Crimean War Letters of Dr. Douglas A. Reid, 1855–1856.* Knoxville: University of Tennessee Press, 1968.

Beadon, R. H. *The Royal Army Service Corps: A History of Transport and Supply in the British Army.* 2 vols.; Cambridge: Cambridge University Press, 1931.

Bedford, William K. R. *Malta and the Knights Hospitallers.* London: Seeley, Service, 1903.

Bedford, William K. R., and Richard Holbeche. *The Order of the Hospital of St. John of Jerusalem.* London: F. E. Robinson, 1902.

Beeston, Joseph Lievesley. *Five Months at Anzac: A Narrative of Personal Experiences of the Officer Commanding the 4th Field Ambulance, Australian Imperial Force.* Sydney: Angus and Robertson, 1916.

Bemrose, John. *Reminiscences of the Second Seminole War.* Gainesville: University Presses of Florida, 1966.

Bergere, Richard, and Thea Bergere. *Automobiles of Yesteryear.* New York: Dodd, Mead, 1962.

Bernhardi, Frederick A. J. *Cavalry in Future Wars.* New York: Dutton, 1906.

Bernhardi, Frederick A. J. *Cavalry in War and Peace.* London: H. Rees, 1910.

Bernhardi, Frederick A. J. *The War of the Future in the Light of the Lessons of the World War.* New York: Appleton, 1921.

Beyer, James C. (ed.). *Wound Ballistics.* Washington, D.C.: Department of the Army, 1962.

Billroth, Theodore. *Chirurgische Briefe aus den kriegs-lazarethen in Weissenburg und Mannkeim 1870.* Berlin: A. Hirschwald, 1872.

Billroth, Theodore. *Historical Studies on the Nature and Treatment of Gunshot Wounds from the 15th Century to the Present Time.* New Haven, Connecticut: Nathan Smith Medical Club, 1953.

Bird, M. Mostyn. *The Errand of Mercy: A History of Ambulance Work upon the Battlefield.* London: Hutchinson, 1913.

Bishop, Denis, and Chris Ellis. *Military Transport of World War I.* New York: Macmillan, 1970.

Blackwood, Alicia. *A Narrative of Personal Experiences and Impressions During a*

Residence on the Bosphorus Throughout the Crimean War. London: Hatchard, 1881.

Blake, Henry Nichols. *Three Years in the Army of the Potomac*. Boston: Lea and Shepherd, 1865.

Blanco, Richard L. *Wellington's Surgeon General, Sir James McGrigor*. Durham, North Carolina: Duke University Press, 1974.

Blenkinsop, Layton John, and J. W. Rainey (eds.). *History of the Great War Based on Official Documents. Veterinary Services*. London: His Majesty's Stationery Office, 1925.

Block, J. *The Future of War: Its Technical, Economic and Political Relations*. Boston: Ginn, 1903.

Bodart, Gaston. *Militär-historisches kriegs-lexikon (1618–1905)*. Leipzig: C. W. Stern, 1908.

Bodart, Gaston, and Vernon L. Kellogg. *Losses of Life in Modern Wars*. Oxford: Clarendon Press, 1916.

Bodfish, Robert W. *A History of Section 647: United States Army Ambulance Service with the French Army*. Worcester, Massachusetts: Stobbs Press, 1919.

Bonham-Carter, V. *Surgeon in the Crimea: The Experiences of George Lawson Recorded in Letters to His Family, 1854–1855*. London: Constable, 1968.

Boudin, Jean. *Contributions a l'hygiène publique*. Paris: Baillière, 1843–65.

Bowditch, Henry I. *Abuse of Army Ambulances*. Boston: n.p., 1863.

Bowerman, Guy Emerson, Jr. *The Compensations of War: The Diary of an Ambulance Driver During the Great War*. Austin: University of Texas Press, 1983.

Bowers, Peter M. *The Fokkers of World War I*. New York: Hobby Helpers Library, 1960.

Brackenbury, Charles B. *European Armaments in 1867*. London: Chapman and Hall, 1867.

Bradley, Amy O. *Back of the Front in France*. Boston: Butterfield, 1918.

Brieger, Gert H. (ed.). *Theory and Practice in American Medicine*. New York: Science History, 1976.

Brinton, John H. *Personal Memoirs of John H. Brinton*. New York: Neal, 1914.

Brogan, Denis W. *The Development of Modern France, 1870–939*. 2 vols.; Gloucester, Massachusetts: Peter Smith, 1970.

Bronsart von Schellendorf, Paul. *The Duties of the General Staff*. London: W. A. H. Hare, 1895.

Brooks, Stewart. *Civil War Medicine*. Springfield, Illinois: Charles C. Thomas, 1966.

Brown, Harvey E. *The Medical Department of the United States Army from 1775 to 1873*. Washington, D.C.: Surgeon General's Office, 1873.

Brumgardt, John R. (ed.). *Civil War Nurse: The Diary and Letters of Hannah Ropes*. Knoxville: University of Tennessee Press, 1980.

Bryan, Julien H. *Ambulance 464: Encore des Blessés*. New York: Macmillan, 1918.

Bucklin, Sophronia E. *In Hospital and Camp: A Woman's Record of Thrilling Incidents Among the Wounded in the Late War*. Philadelphia: J. E. Potter, 1869.

Buswell, Leslie (ed.). *Ambulance No. 10: Personal Letters from the Front*. Boston: Houghton Mifflin, 1916.

Butler, Arthur Graham. *The Australian Army Medical Services in the War of 1914–1918*. 3 vols.; Canberra and Melbourne: Australian War Memorial, 1938–43.

Callan, John. *The Military Laws of the United States Relating to the Army, Volunteers, Militia, and to Bounty Lands and Pensions from the Foundation of the Government to the Year 1863*. Philadelphia: George W. Childs, 1863.

Callwell, Charles Edward. *Experiences of a Dug-out, 1914–1918*. London: Constable, 1920.

Callwell, Charles Edward. *Small Wars. Their Principles and Practice*. 3d ed.; London: Trowbridge and Esher, 1976 [1906].

Cantlie, James. *First Aid to the Injured, Arranged According to the Revised Syllabus of the First Aid Course of the St. John Ambulance Association*. London: St. John Ambulance Association, 1908.

Cantlie, Neil. *A History of the Army Medical Department*. 2 vols.; Edinburgh: Churchill Livingstone, 1974.

Carbery, Anderson Robert Dillon. *The New Zealand Medical Service in the Great War, 1914–1918*. Auckland: Whitcombe and Tombs, 1924.

Carlisle, Robert J. (ed.). *An Account of Bellevue Hospital with a Catalogue of the Medical and Surgical Staff from 1736 to 1894*. New York: Society of the Alumni of Bellevue Hospital, 1893.

Carman, W. Y. *A History of Firearms from Earliest Times to 1914*. New York: St. Martin's Press, 1955.

Carrel, Alexis. *Reflections on Life*. New York: Hawthorn Books, 1953.

Carrel, Alexis, and G. Dehelly. *The Treatment of Infected Wounds*. New York: P. B. Hoeber, 1917.

Cary, Norman Miller, Jr. *The Use of the Motor Vehicle in the United States Army, 1899–1939*. Athens: Unpublished Ph.D. Dissertation, University of Georgia, 1980.

Cash, Philip. *Medical Men at the Seige of Boston*. Philadelphia: American Philosophical Society, 1973.

Catchpool, Corder. *On Two Fronts: Letters of a Conscientious Objector*. New York: Garland, 1972.

Censer, Jane T. (ed.). *The Papers of Frederick Law Olmstead*. Vol. 4. *Defending the Union: The Civil War and the U.S. Sanitary Commission, 1861–1863*. Baltimore: Johns Hopkins University Press, 1986.

Childers, Erskine. *War and the Arme Blanche*. London: E. Arnold, 1910.

Chisolm, John J. *A Manual of Military Surgery, for the Use of Surgeons in the Confederate Army*. Charleston: Evans and Cogswell, 1861.

Church, James R. *The Doctor's Part. What Happens to the Wounded in War*. New York: Appleton, 1918.

Cicero, Marcus Tullius. *Tusculan Disputations*. New York: Putnam, 1927.

Clarke, Edward H., Henry J. Bigelow, Samuel D. Gross, T. Gaillard Thomas, and J. S. Billings. *A Century of American Medicine, 1776–1876*. Brinklow, Maryland: Old Hickory Bookshop, 1876.

Clarkson, Grosvenor B. *Industrial America in the World War*. New York: Houghton Mifflin, 1923.

Clausewitz, Carl von. *On War*. New York: Dutton, 1918.

Clements, Bennett, A. *Memoir of Jonathan Letterman, M.D.* New York: Putnam, 1883.

Clifford, John. *A Good Uniform: The St. John Story*. London: Robert Hale, 1967.

Clifford, John. *For the Service of Mankind: Furley, Lechmere and Duncan, St. John Ambulance Founders*. London: Robert Hale, 1971.

Coffman, Edward M. *The Old Army: A Portrait of the American Army in Peacetime, 1784–1898*. New York: Oxford University Press, 1986.

Coffman, Edward M. *The War to End All Wars: The American Military Experience in World War I*. New York: Oxford University Press, 1968.

Coggins, Jack. *Arms and Equipment of the Civil War*. Garden City, New York: Doubleday, 1962.

Colby, C. B. *Aircraft of World War I: Fighters, Scouts, Bombers, and Observation Planes*. New York: Coward-McCann, 1962.

Colin, J. *The Transformations of War*. Westport, Connecticut: Greenwood Press, 1977 [1912].

Comité des ambulances de la presse. *Les Ambulance de la Presse: Annexes du Ministère de la guerre, pendant le siége et sous la Commune 1870–1871*. Paris: Bailliere, 1872.

Commager, Henry Steele (intro.). *The Official Atlas of the Civil War*. New York: Yoseloff, 1958.

Cooper, Jerry M. *The Army and Civil Disorder: Federal Military Intervention in American Labor Disputes, 1877–1900*. Westport, Connecticut: Greenwood Press, 1980.

Cooperman, Stanley. *World War I and the American Novel*. Baltimore: Johns Hopkins University Press, 1967.

Cope, Zachary. *Florence Nightingale and the Doctors*. London: Museum Press, 1958.

Coplin, William M. L. *American Red Cross Base Hospital No. 38, Organized Under the Auspices of the Jefferson Medical College and Hospital, Stationed at Nantes, France, 1918–1919*. Philadelphia: E. A. Wright, 1923.

Cosmas, Graham A. *An Army for Empire: The United States Army in the Spanish-American War*. Columbia: University of Missouri Press, 1971.

Coulter, E. Merton. *The Confederate States of America, 1861–1865*. Baton Rouge: Louisiana State University Press, 1950.

Cowley, Malcolm. *Exile's Return*. New York: Viking, 1972.

Coyle, Edward R. *Ambulancing on the French Front*. New York: Britton, 1918.

Crile, Grace (ed.). *George Crile: An Autobiography*. Philadelphia: Lippencott, 1947.

Cunningham, Horace H. *Doctors in Gray: The Confederate Medical Service*. Baton Rouge: Louisiana State University Press, 1958.

Cunningham, Horace H. *Field Medical Services at the Battles of Manassas*. Athens: University of Georgia Press, 1968.

Davidson, Henry P. *The American Red Cross in the Great War, 1917–1919*. New York: Russell Sage Foundation, 1943.

Davis, George B. *The War of the Rebellion: A Compilation of the Official Records of the Union and Confederate Armies*. Washington, D.C.: Government Printing Office, 1893.

Dearden, Harold. *Medicine and Duty: A War Diary*. London: Heinemann, 1928.

Dearmer, Mabel. *Letters from a Field Hospital*. New York: Macmillan, 1916.

Delafield, Richard. *Report of the Art of War in Europe in 1854, 1855 and 1856, by Major Richard Delafield, Corps of Engineers, From His Notes and Observations*

Made as a Member of a Military Commission to the Theatre of War in Europe, Under the Orders of the Honorable Jefferson Davis, Secretary of War. Washington, D.C.: George W. Bowman, 1860.

de Tarnowsky, George. *Military Surgery of the Zone of the Advance.*Philadelphia: Lea and Febiger, 1918.

Dible, James Henry. *Napoléon's Surgeon.* London: Heinemann, 1970.

Dodge, Theodore A. *Napoléon: A History of the Art of War, from the Beginning of the French Revolution to the End of the Eighteenth Century, with a Detailed Account of the Wars of the French Revolution.* 4 vols.; Boston: Houghton Mifflin, 1904.

Dooly, William G. *Great Weapons of World War I.* New York: Walter, 1969.

Dunant, Jean-Henri. *Un Souvenir de Solférino.* Geneve: J. Cherbuliez, 1862.

Duncan, Louis C. *The Medical Department of the United States Army in the Civil War.* Gaithersburg, Maryland: Butternut Press, 1985.

Dupuy, George M. *The Stretcher Bearer: A Companion to the R.A.M.C. Training Book, Illustrating the Stretcher Bearer Drill and the Handling and Carrying of Wounded.* London: Oxford University Press, 1915.

Earle, Edward M. *Makers of Modern Strategy: Military Thought From Machiavelli to Hitler.* Princeton, New Jersey: Princeton University Press, 1943.

Edwards, William Sterling. *Alexis Carrel: Visionary Surgeon.* Springfield, Illinois: Charles C. Thomas, 1974.

Eggenhofer, Nick. *Wagons, Mules and Men: How the Frontier Moved West.* New York: Hastings House, 1961.

Ellis, John. *Eye-Deep in Hell: Trench Warfare in World War I.* New York: Pantheon, 1976.

Emergency War Medicine. Washington, D.C.: Government Printing Office, 1975.

Encyclopaedia Britannica: A Dictionary of Arts, Sciences and General Literature. 25 vols.; 9th ed.; Boston: Little, Brown, 1875–89.

Engle, Eloise. *Medic: America's Medical Soldiers, Sailors and Airmen in Peace and War.* New York: John Day, 1967.

English Combatant. *Battle-Fields of the South, from Bull Run to Fredericksburg; With Sketches of Confederate Commanders, and Gossip of the Camps.* New York: John Bradburn, 1864.

Evans, Thomas W. *La commission sanitaire des États-Unis, son origine, son organisation et ses résultats, avec une notice sur les hôpitaux militaires aux États-Unis et sur la réforme sanitaire dans les armees européennes.* Paris: É. Dentu, 1865.

Evans, Thomas W. *History of the American Ambulance Established in Paris During the Siege of 1870–1871, Together with the Details of Its Methods and Its Work.* London: S. Low, Marston, Low and Searle, 1873.

Evans, Thomas W. *History and Description of an Ambulance Wagon, Constructed in Accordance with Plans Furnished by the Writer.* Paris: E. Briere, 1868.

Evatt, George J. H. *Ambulance Organization, Equipment, and Transport.* London: William Clowes, 1886.

Evatt, George J. H. *On the Organization and Duties of the Bearer Company of the Medical Corps in War.* London: Ballantyne, Hanson, 1886.

Evatt, George J. H. *Suggestions for the Reorganization of the Volunteer Medical Service and for the Utilization of Voluntary Medical Aid in War.* Woolwich: F. J. Cattermole, 1885.

Falls, Cyril B. *The Art of War: From the Age of Napoléon to the Present Day*. New York: Oxford University Press, 1961.

Falls, Cyril B. *The First World War*. London: Longmans, Green, 1960.

Falls, Cyril B. *A Hundred Years of War, 1850–1950*. New York: Collier Books, 1962.

Falls, Cyril B. *Military Operations, France and Belgium, 1917*. 3 vols.; London: Macmillan, 1940–48.

Falls, Cyril B., and Edmund Blunden (comps.). *The War, 1914–18: A Booklist*. London: Published by the Reader, 1929.

Farrow, Edward S. *Gas Warfare*. New York: Dutton, 1920.

Fatout, Paul (ed.). *Letters of a Civil War Surgeon*. West Lafayette, Indiana: Purdue University Research Foundation, 1961.

Fauntleroy, Archibald Magill. *Report on the Medico-Military Aspects of the European War: From Observations Taken Behind the Allied Armies in France*. Washington, D.C.: Government Printing Office, 1915.

Fenton, Norman. *Shell Shock and Its Aftermath*. St. Louis: C. V. Mosby, 1926.

Fergusson, William. *A System of Practical Surgery*. Philadelphia: Lee and Blanchard, 1845.

Fletcher, N. Corbet. *The St. John Ambulance Association: Its History, and Its Part in the Ambulance Movement*. London: St. John Ambulance Association, 1929.

Fletcher, William A. *Rebel Private Front and Rear*. Austin: University of Texas Press, 1954.

Florez, C. de. *"No. 6": A Few Pages from the Diary of an Ambulance Driver*. New York: Dutton, 1918.

Forbes, Archibald. *My Experiences of the War Between France and Germany*. 2 vols.; London: Hurst and Blackett, 1871.

Forman, Jacob G. *The Western Sanitary Commission. A Sketch of Its Origin, History, Labors for the Sick and Wounded of the Western Armies, and Aid Given to Freedmen and Union Refugees, with Incidents of Hospital Life*. St. Louis: R. P. Studley, 1864.

Fortescue, John, and R. H. Beadon. *The Royal Army Service Corps: A History of Transport and Supply in the British Army*. 2 vols.; Cambridge: Cambridge University Press, 1930–31.

Frank, Jacob. *The Fate of Our Wounded in the Next War*. Chicago: n.p., 1916.

Freeman, N. N. *A Soldier in the Philippines*. New York: F. Tennyson Neely, 1901.

Fremantle, Arthur James. *Three Months in the Southern States, April–June, 1863*. London: William Blackwood, 1864.

Fries, Amos A., and Clarence J. West. *Chemical Warfare*. New York: McGraw Hill, 1921.

Fuller, Stephen M. *Marines in the Dominican Republic, 1916–1924*. Washington, D.C.: Government Printing Office, 1974.

Funston, Frederick. *Memoirs of Two Wars: Cuban and Philippine Experiences*. New York: Scribner, 1914.

Furley, Sir John. *In Peace and War: Autobiographical Sketches*. London: Smith, Elder, 1905.

Futrell, Robert F. *Development of Aeromedical Evacuation in the U.S.A.F., 1909–1960*. United States Air Force Historical Division: Research Studies Institute Air University, 1960.

Gagnebin, Bernard. *Encounter with Henry Dunant*. Geneva: Georg, 1963.

Gaines, Ruth L. *Helping France: The Red Cross in the Devastated Area*. New York: Dutton, 1919.

Ganoe, William A. *The History of the United States Army*. Ashton, Maryland: Eric Lundberg, 1964.

Garrison, Fielding H. *An Introduction to the History of Medicine*. 4th ed.; Philadelphia: Saunders, 1929.

Garrison, Fielding H. *Notes on the History of Military Medicine*. Washington, D.C.: Association of Military Surgery, 1922.

Gask, George. *Essays in the History of Medicine*. London: Butterworth, 1950.

Gates, John Morgan. *Schoolbooks and Krags: The United States Army in the Philippines, 1898–1902*. Westport, Connecticut: Greenwood Press, 1973.

Geller, L. D. *The American Field Service Archives of World War I, 1914–1917*. Westport, Connecticut: Greenwood Press, 1989.

Gibbs, P. *Crimean Blunder*. New York: Holt, Rinehart and Winston, 1960.

Gibson, John M. *Soldier in White: The Life of General George Miller Sternberg*. Durham, North Carolina: Duke University Press, 1958.

Giddings, Luther. *Sketches of the Campaign in Northern Mexico in Eighteen Hundred Forty-six and Seven*. New York: Putnam, 1853.

Gilchrist, H. L. *Chemical Warfare: Medical Aspects; Their History; Classification; Symptoms Produced; Pathology and Treatment*. Washington, D.C.: Government Printing Office, 1922.

Gilchrist, H. L. *A Comparative Study of Warfare Gases: Their History, Description and Medical Aspects*. Washington, D.C.: Government Printing Office, 1925.

Gilchrist, H. L. *A Comparative Study of World War Casualties from Gas and Other Weapons*. Washington, D.C.: Government Printing Office, 1928.

Gilchrist, H. L. *Report on the After Effects of Warfare Gases*. Washington, D.C.: Chemical Warfare Service, 1923.

Gillett, Mary C. *The Army Medical Department, 1775–1818*. Washington, D.C.: Government Printing Office, 1981.

Gillett, Mary C. *The Army Medical Department, 1818–1865*. Washington, D.C.: Center for Military History, 1987.

Gleason, Arthur H. *With the First War Ambulance in Belgium: Young Hilda at the Wars*. New York: A. L. Burt, 1915.

Gleaves, Albert. *Life and Letters of Rear Admiral Stephen B. Luce*. New York: Putnam, 1925.

Gordon, Charles A. *Army Hygiene*. London: Churchill, 1866.

Gordon, Charles A. *Experiences of an Army Surgeon in India*. London: Bailliere, Tindall and Cox, 1872.

Gordon, Charles A. *Lessons on Hygiene and Surgery from the Franco-Prussian War*. London: Bailliere, Tindall and Cox, 1873.

Grace, William. *The Army Surgeon's Manual*. 2d ed.; New York: Bailliere, 1865.

Grant, James Hope. *Incidents in the China War of 1860*. Edinburgh: William Blackwood, 1875.

Grant, James Hope. *Incidents in the Sepoy War, 1857–58*. London: William Blackwood, 1873.

Grant, John H. *Registrar of Hospital Stewards, U.S. Army, January 1, 1883, with Brief History of Their Organization*. San Antonio, Texas: Shepard Brothers, 1883.

Grant, Ulysses S. *Personal Memoirs*. 2 vols.; New York: Charles L. Webster, 1886.

Great Britain. Army Medical Services. *Medical and Surgical History of the British Army Which Served in Turkey and the Crimea During the War Against Russia in the Years 1854–55–56.* 2 vols.; London: Harrison, 1858.

Great Britain. Medical Research Committee. *An Atlas of Gas Poisoning.* Great Britain: American Red Cross, 1918.

Greenleaf, Charles R. *A Manual for the Medical Officers of the United States Army.* Philadelphia: Lippincott, 1864.

Grey, Elizabeth. *The Noise from the Drums: W. H. Russell Reports from the Crimea.* London: Longmans, 1971.

Groves, Ernest W. *Gunshot Injuries of Bones.* London: Frowde, 1915.

Guerra, Francisco. *American Medical Bibliography 1639–1783.* New York: Harper, 1982.

Gumpert, Martin. *Dunant: The Story of the Red Cross.* New York: Oxford University Press, 1938.

Gurlt, Ernst J. *Abbildungen zur krankenpflege im felde aufgrund der Internationalen ausstellung der hilfs-vereine für verwundete zu Paris im jahre 1867, und mit benutzung der besten vorhandenen modelle.* Berlin: T. C. F. Enslin, 1868.

Gurlt, Ernst J. *Militär-chirurgische Fragmente.* Berlin: Hirschwald, 1864.

Guthrie, Douglas. *A History of Medicine.* London: Lippincott, 1946.

Guthrie, George James. *Commentaries on the Surgery of the War in Portugal, Spain, France and the Netherlands, from the Battle of Rolica, in 1808, to That of Waterloo, in 1815: With Additions Relating to Those in the Crimea in 1854–55.* London: Henry Renshaw, 1855.

Guthrie, George James. *On Gunshot Wounds of the Extremities Requiring the Different Operations of Amputation.* London: Longman, 1815.

Haber, Ludwig Fritz. *The Chemical Industry During the Nineteenth Century.* Oxford: Clarendon Press, 1958.

Haber, Ludwig Fritz. *The Chemical Industry, 1900–1930.* Oxford: Clarendon Press, 1971.

Haber, Ludwig Fritz. *The Poisonous Cloud: Chemical Warfare in the First World War.* New York: Oxford University Press, 1986.

Hagan, Kenneth J., and William R. Roberts (eds.). *Against All Enemies: Interpretations of American Military History from Colonial Times to the Present.* Westport, Connecticut: Greenwood Press, 1986.

Hager, Philip E. *The Novels of World War I: An Annotated Bibliography.* New York: Garland, 1981.

Haig, Douglas. *Cavalry Studies: Strategical and Tactical.* London: H. Rees, 1907.

Haigh, R. H., and P. W. Turner (eds.). *The Long Carry: The Journal of Stretcher-Bearer Frank Dunham, 1916–18.* New York: Pergamon, 1970.

Hamby, Wallace B. *Ambroise Paré, Surgeon of the Renaissance.* St. Louis: Warren H. Green, 1967.

Hamilton, Frank Hastings. *A Practical Treatise on Military Surgery and Hygiene.* New York: Bailliere, 1861.

Hamilton, Frank Hastings. *Surgical Memoirs of the War of the Rebellion.* New York: U.S. Sanitary Commission, 1870.

Hammond, William A. *A Statement of the Causes Which Led to the Dismissal of Surgeon-General William A. Hammond from the Army.* New York: n.p., 1864.

Hammond, William A. *A Treatise on Hygiene with Special Reference to the Military Service*. Philadelphia: Lippincott, 1863.

Harris, Elisha. *The United States Sanitary Commission*. Boston: Crosby and Nichols, 1864.

Harrison, Carter Henry. *With the American Red Cross in France, 1918–1919*. Chicago: Ralph Fletcher Seymour, 1947.

Harrison, Reginald. *The Ambulance in Civil Life on Land and Sea*. London: Bale and Danielsson, 1902.

Harrison, Reginald. *The Use of the Ambulance in Civil Practice*. Liverpool: n.p., 1881.

Heizmann, Charles L. *Provisional Manual of Instruction*. Washington, D.C.: Government Printing Office, 1888.

Hemingway, Ernest. *A Farwell to Arms*. New York: Modern Library, 1929.

Hennessy, Juliette. *The United States Army Air Arm, April 1861 to April 1917*. Air University: U.S.A.F. Historical Studies No. 98, 1958.

Henniker, Colonel A. M. (comp.). *Transportation on the Western Front, 1914–1918*. London: His Majesty's Stationery Office, 1937.

Hicks, John W. *The Theory of the Rifle and Rifle Shooting. An Elementary Treatise on the Scientific Principles of the Smallarm and Its Functions*. London: Griffin, 1919.

History of Ambulance Company Number 139. Kansas City, Missouri: E. R. Callender, 1919.

The History of U.S. Army Base Hospital No. 6 and Its Part in the American Expeditionary Forces, 1917–1918. Boston: Thomas Todd, 1924.

Holland, Sir Henry. *Recollections of Past Life*. London: Longmans, Green, 1872.

Homer. *Iliad*. London: Macmillan, 1886.

Hooker, Dorothy. *The Trenches: Fighting on the Western Front in World War I*. New York: Putnam, 1978.

Horne, Alistair. *The Price of Glory: Verdun 1916*. London: Macmillan, 1962.

Howard, Michael. *The Franco-Prussian War: The German Invasion of France, 1870–1871*. London: Methuen, 1967.

Howard, Michael (ed.). *The Theory and Practice of War*. Bloomington: Indiana University Press, 1975.

Howe, Mark A. De Wolfe (ed.). *The Harvard Volunteers in Europe: Personal Records of the Experience in Military, Ambulance, and Hospital Service*. Cambridge, Massachusetts: Harvard University Press, 1916.

Howie-Willis, Ian. *A Century for Australia: St. John Ambulance in Australia, 1883–1983*. Canberra: Priory of the Order of St. John in Australia, 1983.

Howland, Charles R. *A Military History of the World War*. 2 vols.; Fort Leavenworth, Kansas: General Service Schools, 1923.

Hume, Edgar E. *Medical Work of the Knights Hospitallers of St. John of Jerusalem*. Baltimore: Johns Hopkins University Press, 1940.

Huntington, David L., and George A. Otis. *Hospital of Medical Department, United States Army. No. 6. Description of the U.S. Army Medical Transport Cart, Model of 1876*. Philadelphia: International Exhibition, 1876.

Hurst, Arthur F. *Medical Diseases of the War*. London: Edward Arnold, 1918.

Huston, James A. *The Sinews of War: Army Logistics, 1775–1953*. Washington, D.C.: Office of the Chief of Military History, 1966.

Hutchinson, Woods. *The Doctor in War*. Boston: Houghton Mifflin, 1918.

Hutton, George A. *Reminiscences in the Life of Surgeon-Major George A. Hutton*. London: H. K. Lewis, 1907.

Ireland, M. W. (ed.). *The Medical Department of the United States Army in the World War, 1917–1918*. 15 vols.; Washington, D.C.: Government Printing Office, 1921–29.

Jackson, Aubrey Joseph. *De Havilland Aircraft Since 1909*. London: Putnam, 1987.

James, Henry. *Within the Rim, and Other Essays, 1914–1915*. London: W. Collins, 1918.

Johnson, Charles B. *Muskets and Medicine, or Army Life in the Sixties*. Philadelphia: F. A. Davis, 1917.

Johnson, Edward C. *Marine Corps Aviation: The Early Years, 1912–1940*. Washington, D.C.: Government Printing Office, 1977.

Johnson, L. W. *Eight Hundred Miles in an Ambulance*. Philadelphia:Lippincott, 1889.

Johnson, Thomas (trans.). *The Workes of that Famous Chirurgion Ambrose Parey* New York: Milford House, 1968 [1634].

Judd, James R. *With the American Ambulance in France*. Honolulu: Star-Bulletin Press, 1919.

Junger, Ernst. *Copse 125: A Chronicle from the Trench Warfare of 1918*. London: Chatto and Windus, 1930.

Kaletzki, Charles H. (ed.). *Official History: U.S.A. Base Hospital No. 31 of Youngstown, Ohio, and Hospital Unit "G" of Syracuse University* Syracuse, New York: Craftsmen Press, 1918.

Kane, Joseph N. *Famous First Facts*. New York: Wilson, 1964.

Karsten, Peter. *The Naval Aristocracy: The Golden Age of Annapolis and the Emergence of Modern American Navalism*. New York: Free Press, 1972.

Karsten, Peter (ed.). *The Military in America: From the Colonial Era to the Present*. New York: Free Press, 1980.

Keen, W. W. *The Treatment of War Wounds*. Philadelphia: Saunders, 1917.

Kernodle, Portia B. *The Red Cross Nurse in Action, 1882–1948*. New York: Harper, 1949.

Kimball, Marcia Brace. *A Soldier-Doctor of Our Army: James P. Kimball*. Boston: Houghton Mifflin, 1917.

Klein, Felix. *Diary of a French Army Chaplain*. London: A. Melrose, 1917.

Knight, Oliver. *Life and Manners in the Frontier Army*. Norman: University of Oklahoma Press, 1978.

L., R. A. *Letters of a Canadian Stretcher Bearer*. Boston: Little, Brown, 1917.

A Lady Volunteer [Fanny Taylor]. *Eastern Hospitals and English Nurses: The Narrative of Twelve Months' Experience in the Hospitals of Koulali and Scutari*. 2 vols.; London: Hurst and Blackett, 1856.

LaGarde, Louis A. *Gunshot Injuries: How They Are Inflicted, Their Complications and Treatment*. 2d ed.; New York: William Wood, 1916.

Larrey, Dominque-Jean. *Dissertation sur les amputations des membres à la suite des coups de feu, étayée de plusieurs observations*. Paris: n.p., 1803.

Larrey, Dominque-Jean. *Mémoires de chirurgie militaire, et campagnes*. 4 vols.; Paris: J. Smith, 1812–17.

Larrey, Dominque-Jean. *Memoirs of Military Surgery. Containing the Practice of the*

French Military Surgeons During the Principal Campaigns of the Late War. London: Cox, 1815.

Larrey, Dominque-Jean. *Observations on Wounds and Their Complications by Erysipelas, Gangrene and Tetanus, and on the Principal Diseases and Injuries of the Head, Ear and Eye*. Philadelphia: Key, Mielke and Biddle, 1832.

Larrey, Dominque-Jean. *Surgical Essays*. Baltimore: N. G. Maxwell, 1823.

Larrey, Dominque-Jean. *Surgical Memoirs of the Campaigns of Russia, Germany and France*. Philadelphia: Carey and Lea, 1832.

Leech, Margaret. *In the Days of McKinley*. New York: Harper, 1959.

Leed, Eric J. *No Man's Land: Combat and Identity in World War I*. Cambridge: Cambridge University Press, 1979.

Lefebure, Victor. *The Riddle of the Rhine: Chemical Strategy in Peace and War*. New York: Dutton, 1923.

Legouest, Venant A. L. *Traité de chirurgie d'armée*. Paris: Bailliere, 1863.

Leng, William St. Q. *S.S.A. 10. Notes on the Work of a British Volunteer Ambulance Convoy with the 2nd French Army*. Sheffield: Leng, 1918.

Leonard, Thomas E. *Above the Battle: War-Making in America from Appomattox to Versailles*. New York: Oxford University Press, 1978.

Letterman, Jonathan. *Medical Recollections of the Army of the Potomac*. New York: Appleton, 1866.

Lewis, Emanuel R. *Seacoast Fortifications of the United States: An Introductory History*. Washington, D.C.: Smithsonian Institute Press, 1970.

Libby, Violet K. *Henry Dunant: Prophet of Peace*. New York: Pagent Press, 1964.

Linn, Brian McAllister. *The U.S. Army and Counterinsurgency in the Philippine War, 1899–1902*. Chapel Hill: University of North Carolina Press, 1989.

Livermore, Mary A. *My Story of the War: A Woman's Narrative of Four Years' Personal Experience as Nurse in the Union Army, and in Relief Work at Home, in Hospitals, Camps, and at the Front, During the War of the Rebellion*. Hartford, Connecticut: A. D. Worthington, 1889.

Livermore, Thomas L. *Numbers and Losses in the Civil War in America, 1861–1865*. Boston: Houghton Mifflin, 1901.

Longmore, Thomas. *Amputation: An Historical Sketch*. Glasgow: Bell and Bain, 1876.

Longmore, Thomas. *On the Geneva Convention of August the 22nd, 1864, with Some Account of the National Committees Formed for Aiding in Ameliorating the Condition of the Sick and Wounded of Armies in Time of War*. London: n.p., 1866.

Longmore, Thomas. *Gunshot Injuries: Their History, Characteristic Features, Complications, and General Treatment; with Statistics Concerning Them as They Are Met with in Warfare*. London: Longmans, Green, 1877.

Longmore, Thomas. *A Manual of Ambulance Transport*. London: Harrison, 1893.

Longmore, Thomas. *The Sanitary Contrasts of the British and French Armies During the Crimean War*. London: C. Griffin, 1883.

Longmore, Thomas. *A Treatise on the Transport of Sick and Wounded Troops*. London: William Clowes, 1869.

Lord, Francis A. *They Fought for the Union*. Harrisburg, Pennsylvania: Stackpole, 1960.

Lord, William B., and Thomas Baines. *Shifts and Expedients of Camp Life, Travel, and Exploration*. London: Sheldon, 1871.

Lowenfels, Walter (ed.). *Walt Whitman's Civil War*. New York: Knopf, 1961.

Luvaas, Jay (ed. and trans.). *Frederick the Great on the Art of War*. New York: Free Press, 1966.

MacCormac, William. *Notes and Recollections of an Ambulance Surgeon, Being an Account of Work Done Under the Red Cross During the Campaign of 1870*. London: J. and A. Churchill, 1871.

MacLeod, George H. B. *War in the Crimea, with Remarks on the Treatment of Gunshot Wounds*. Philadelphia: Lippincott, 1862.

Macpherson, William G. (ed.). *History of the Great War Based on Official Documents*. 12 vols.; London: His Majesty's Stationery Office, 1921–31.

McClellan, George B. *Army of the Potomac: Report, August 4, 1863, with an Account of the Campaign in Western Virginia*. New York: Sheldon, 1864.

McClellan, George B. *McClellan's Own Story: The War for the Union, the Soldiers Who Fought It, the Civilians Who Directed It, and His Relations to It and to Them*. New York: Charles L. Webster, 1886.

McClellan, George B. *Report of the Secretary of War, Communicating the Report of Captain George B. McClellan, One of the Officers Sent to the Seat of War in Europe in 1855 and 1856*. Washington, D.C.: Nicholson, 1857.

McElderry, Henry. *Descriptions of the Models of Hospital Cars, From the U.S. Army Medical Museum, Washington, D.C.* New Orleans: World's Industrial and Cotton Centennial Exposition, 1884–85.

McPherson, Thomas A. *American Funeral Cars and Ambulances Since 1900*. Glen Ellyn, Illinois: Cresline, 1973.

Mahan, Alfred T. *The Influence of Sea Power upon the French Revolution and Empire, 1793–1812*. Boston: Little, Brown, 1892.

Mahan, Alfred T. *The Influence of Sea Power upon History, 1660–1783*. Boston: Little, Brown, 1890.

Mahan, Alfred T. *Sea Power in Its Relations to the War of 1812*. Boston: Little, Brown, 1905.

Majno, Guido. *The Healing Hand: Man and Wound in the Ancient World*. Cambridge, Massachusetts: Harvard University Press, 1975.

Major, Ralph H. *Fatal Partners: War and Disease*. New York: Doubleday, Dozan, 1941.

Malgaigne, Joseph Francois. *Surgery and Ambroise Paré*. Norman: University of Oklahoma Press, 1965.

Mann, James. *Medical Sketches of the Campaigns of 1812–13–14. To Which Are Added, Surgical Cases; Observations on Military Hospitals; and Flying Hospitals Attached to a Moving Army*. Dedham, Massachusetts: H. Mann, 1816.

Manning, Van H. *War Gas Investigations*. Washington, D.C.: Government Printing Office, 1919.

Marcy, Randolph B. *The Prairie Traveler. A Hand-book for Overland Expeditions*. New York: Harper, 1859.

Marks, Geoffrey, and William K. Beatty. *The Story of Medicine in America*. New York: Scribner, 1973.

Martin, Kingsley. *The Triumph of Lord Palmerston: A Study of Public Opinion in England Before the Crimean War*. London: Allen and Unwin, 1924.

Maude, Frederic N. *Cavalry Versus Infantry*. Kansas City, Missouri: Hudson-Kimberly, 1896.

Maurice, F. *The System of Field Manoeuvres Best Adapted for Enabling Our Troops To Meet a Continental Army.* 2d ed.; London: William Blackwood, 1872.

Maxwell, William Quentin. *Lincoln's Fifth Wheel: The Political History of the United States Sanitary Commission.* New York: Longmans, Green, 1956.

A Member of the Unit. *The Story of United States Army Base Hospital No. 5.* Cambridge: Cambridge University Press, 1919.

Middlebrook, Martin. *The First Day on the Somme, 1 July 1916.* New York: Norton, 1972.

Miller, Francis T. (ed.). *The Photographic History of the Civil War.* 10 vols.; New York: Review of Reviews, 1911.

Miller, Stewart C. *"Benevolent Assimilation": The American Conquest of the Philippines, 1899–1903.* New Haven, Connecticut: Yale University Press, 1982.

Millett, Alan R., and Peter Maslowski. *For the Common Defense: A Military History of the United States of America.* New York: Free Press, 1984.

Mitchell, Silas Weir. *The Early History of Instrumental Precision in Medicine.* New Haven, Connecticut: Tuttle, Morehouse and Taylor, 1892.

Mitchell, William. *Memories of World War I: "From Start to Finish of Our Greatest War."* New York: Random House, 1960.

Mitra, Siddha M. *The Life and Letters of Sir John Hall.* New York: Longmans, Green, 1911.

Moore, George A. *The Birth and Early Days of Our Ambulance Trains in France, August, 1914, to April, 1915.* London: John Bale Sons and Danielsson, 1922.

Morrison, John F., and Edward L. Munson. *A Study in Troop Leading and Management of the Sanitary Service in War.* Menasha, Wisconsin: George Banta, 1918.

Morse, Edward Wilson. *The Vanguard of American Volunteers in the Fighting Lines and in Humanitarian Service, August, 1914–April, 1917.* New York: Scribner, 1918.

Moss, James A. *Trench Warfare.* Menasha, Wisconsin: George Banta, 1917.

Mottier, Georgette. *L'Ambulance du docteur Alexis Carrel telle que l'ont connue celles qui soignerent les blessés, 1914–1919.* Lausanne: Payot, 1977.

Munson, Edward L. *The Management of Men: A Handbook on the Systematic Development of Morale and the Control of Human Behavior.* New York: Henry Holt, 1921.

Munson, Edward L. *The Principles of Sanitary Tactics: A Handbook on the Use of Medical Department Detachments and Organizations in Campaign.* Menasha, Wisconsin: George Banta, 1917.

Munson, Edward L. *The Theory and Practice of Military Hygiene.* New York: William Wood, 1901.

Myers, George G. T. *Strategy.* Washington, D.C.: Bryon S. Adams, 1928.

Nenninger, Timothy K. *The Leavenworth Schools and the Old Army: Education, Professionalism, and the Officer Corps of the United States Army, 1881–1918.* Westport, Connecticut: Greenwood Press, 1978.

Neudörfer, Ignaz Joseph. *Handbuch der Kriegschirurgie.* Leipzig: Vogel, 1864–67.

Nichols, Francis H. *The New York Ambulance Service.* New York: n.p., 1901.

Orcutt, Philip Dana. *The White Road of Mystery: The Note-book of an American Ambulancier.* New York: John Lane, 1918.

Otis, George A. *A Report on a Plan for Transporting Wounded Soldiers by Railway in*

Time of War, with Descriptions of Various Methods Employed for This Purpose on Different Occasions. Washington, D.C.: War Department, Surgeon General's Office, 1875.

Otis, George A. *A Report to the Surgeon General on the Transport of Sick and Wounded by Pack Animals*. Washington, D.C.: Government Printing Office, 1877.

Packard, Francis R. *History of Medicine in the United States*. 2 vols.; New York: Hafner, 1963.

Paré, Ambroise. *The Workes of that Famous Chirurgion Ambrose Parey*. London: Thomas Cotes and R. Young, 1634 [facsimile; New York: Milford House, 1968].

Parkman, Francis. *California and Oregon Trail: Being Sketches of Prairie and Rocky Mountain Life*. New York: Putnam, 1849.

Parkman, Francis. *History of the Conspiracy of Pontiac, and the War of the North American Tribes Against the English Colonies After the Conquest of Canada*. Boston: Little, Brown, 1851.

Pember, Phoebe Yates. *A Southern Woman's Story: Life in Confederate Richmond*. Jackson, Tennessee: McCowat-Mercer Press, 1959.

Penrose, Harold. *British Aviation: The Pioneer Years 1903–1914*. London: Putnam, 1967.

Percy, Pierre François. *Journal des campagnes du Baron Percy: chirurgien en chef de la grande armée (1754–1825)*. Paris: Plon-Nourrit, 1904.

Peterson, H. L. *The Book of the Continental Soldier*. Harrisburg, Pennsylvania: Promontory Press, 1968.

Phistener, Frederick. *Statistical Record of the Armies of the United States*. New York: Scribner, 1907.

Pincoffs, Peter. *Experiences of a Civilian in Eastern Military Hospitals*. London: William and Norgate, 1857.

Plumridge, John H. *Hospital Ships and Ambulance Trains*. London: Seeley, Service, 1975.

Poling, Daniel A. *Huts in Hell*. Boston: Christian Endeavor World, 1918.

Pratt, Edwin A. *The Rise of Rail Power in War and Conquest, 1833–1914*. London: P. S. King, 1915.

Prentiss, Augustin M. *Chemicals in War: A Treatise on Chemical Warfare*. New York: McGraw-Hill, 1937.

Puddy, Eric. *A Short History of the Order of the Hospital of St. John of Jerusalem in Norfolk, from Knights Hospitallers, 1163, to Ambulance Brigade, 1961*. Dereham: Starling, 1961.

Quimby, Robert S. *The Background of Napoleonic Warfare: The Theory of Military Tactics in Eighteenth-Century France*. New York: AMS Press, 1968.

Randall, James G. *The Civil War and Reconstruction*. Boston: D.C. Heath, 1937.

Randall, James G., and David Donald. *The Divided Union*. Boston: Little, Brown, 1961.

Reed, William H. *Hospital Life in the Army of the Potomac*. Boston: William V. Spencer, 1866.

Reid, Douglas A. *Memories of the Crimean War*. London: St. Catherine Press, 1911.

Remak, Joachim. *The Origins of World War I, 1871–1914*. New York: Holt, Rinehart and Winston, 1967.

Remantle, T. F. *The Book of the Rifle*. New York: Longmans, Green, 1901.

Remarque, Erich. *All Quiet on the Western Front*. Boston: Little, Brown, 1921.

Report of the British National Society To Aid Sick and Wounded in War, Franco-German War. London: n.p., 1871.

Report upon the State of the Hospitals of the British Army in the Crimea and Scutari. London: Eyre and Spottiswood, 1855.

Richardson, Robert G. *Larrey: Surgeon to Napoléon's Imperial Guard*. London: John Murray, 1974.

Rickey, Don, Jr. *Forty Miles a Day on Beans and Hay: The Enlisted Soldier Fighting the Indian Wars*. Norman: University of Oklahoma Press, 1963.

Riddell, John S. *A Manual of Ambulance*. London: Griffin, 1894.

Risch, Erna. *Quartermaster Support of the Army: A History of the Corps, 1775–1939*. Washington, D.C.: Quartermaster Historian's Office, Office of the Quartermaster General, 1962.

Roberts, Richard Lawton. *Illustrated Lectures on Ambulance Work*. London: Lewis, 1888.

Rogers, H. C. B. *The Mounted Troops of the British Army, 1066–1945*. London: Seeley, Service, 1959.

Rothenberg, Gunther E. *The Art of Warfare in the Age of Napoléon*. London: B. T. Batsford, 1977.

Rund, Douglas A., and Tondra S. Rausch. *Triage*. St. Louis: Mosby, 1981.

Rundle, Henry. *With the Red Cross in the Franco-German War*. London: Werner Laurie, 1911.

Russell, William H. *The British Expedition to the Crimea*. New York: G. Routledge, 1858.

Russell, William H. *Despatches from the Crimea, 1854–1856*. London: Deutsch, 1966.

Ryan, Charles Edward. *With an Ambulance During the Franco-German War, Personal Experiences and Adventures with Both Armies, 1870–1871*. New York: Scribner, 1896.

Ryan, Charles S. *Under the Red Crescent: Adventures of an English Surgeon with the Turkish Army at Plevna and Erzerum, 1877–1878*. New York: Scribner, 1897.

Scarborough, John. *Roman Medicine*. Ithaca, New York: Cornell University Press, 1969.

Schaffer, Ronald. *The United States in World War I: A Selected Bibliography*. Santa Barbara, California: Clio Books, 1978.

Schott, Joseph L. *The Ordeal of Samar*. Indianapolis: Bobbs-Merrill, 1964.

Scott, Winfield. *General Regulations for the Army: Or, Military Institutes*. Washington, D.C.: n.p., 1825.

Senn, Nicholas. *Medico-Surgical Aspects of the Spanish-American War*. Chicago: American Medical Association Press, 1900.

Senn, Nicholas. *War Correspondence*. Chicago: American Medical Association Press, 1899.

Sexton, William T. *Soldiers in the Sun: An Adventure in Imperialism*. Harrisburg, Pennsylvania: Military Services, 1939.

Shannon, Fred A. *The Organization and Administration of the Union Army, 1861–1865*. 2 vols.; Gloucester, Massachusetts: Peter Smith, 1965.

Sharpe, Major General Henry G. *The Quartermaster Corps in the Year 1917 in the World War*. New York: Century, 1921.

Shaw, Colonel G. C. *Supply in Modern War*. London: Faber and Faber, 1938.

Shepherd, John A. *Spencer Wells: The Life and Work of a Victorian Surgeon*. Edinburgh: E. and S. Livingstone, 1965.

Shepherd, Peter. *Handbook Describing Aids for Cases of Injuries or Sudden Illness*. London: Army and Navy Cooperative Society, 1878.

Shepperd, Gilbert A. *Arms and Armour, 1660–1918*. New York: Crowell, 1972.

Shipley, A. E. *The Minor Horrors of War*. 3d ed.; London: Smith, Elder, 1916.

Shryock, Richard H. *The Development of Modern Medicine: An Interpretation of the Social and Scientific Factors Involved*. New York: Knopf, 1947.

Shryock, Richard H. *Medicine in America: Historical Essays*. Baltimore: Johns Hopkins University Press, 1966.

Smart, Charles. *Handbook for the Hospital Corps of the U.S. Army and State Military Forces*. New York: William Wood, 1889.

Smith, George W. *Medicines for the Union Army*. Madison, Wisconsin: American Institute of the History of Pharmacy, 1962.

Smith, J. S. *Trench Warfare: A Manual for Officers and Men*. New York: Dutton, 1917.

Southard, E. E. *Shell-Shock and Other Neuropsychiatric Problems in 589 Case Histories from the War Literature, 1914–1918*. Boston: W. M. Leonard, 1919.

Spaulding, Oliver L., Jr., Hoffman Nickerson, and John W. Wright. *Warfare: A Study of Military Methods from the Earliest Times*. New York: Harcourt, Brace, 1925.

Speedy, John Clark, III. *From Mules to Motors: Development of Maintenance Doctrine for Motor Vehicles by the U.S. Army, 1895–1917*. Durham: Unpublished Master's Thesis, Duke University, 1973.

Stackpole, Edward J. *Drama on the Rappahannock: The Fredericksburg Campaign*. Harrisburg, Pennsylvania: Military Service, 1957.

Statham, Sherrard F. *On the Fractures of Bones Occurring in Gun-Shot Injuries*. London: Trubner, 1860.

Steiner, Paul E. *Disease in the Civil War: Natural Biological Warfare in 1861–65*. Springfield, Illinois: Charles C. Thomas, 1968.

Steiner, Paul E. *Physician-Generals in the Civil War: A Study in Nineteenth Century American Medicine*. Springfield, Illinois: Charles C. Thomas, 1966.

Sternberg, George M. *Sanitary Lessons of the War, and Other Papers*. Washington, D.C.: Byron S. Adams, 1912.

Stevenson, William F. *Wounds in War: The Mechanism of Their Production and Their Treatment*. New York: William Wood, 1898.

Stewart, Isabel, and Anne L. Austin. *A History of Nursing from Ancient to Modern Times: A World View*. New York: Putnam, 1962.

Stewart, Miller J. *Moving the Wounded: Litters, Cacolets and Ambulance Wagons, U.S. Army, 1776–1876*. Fort Collins, Colorado: Old Army Press, 1979.

Stillé, Charles J. *History of the United States Sanitary Commission; Being the General Report of Its Work During the War of the Rebellion*. Philadelphia: Lippincott, 1866.

The Story of U.S. Army Base Hospital No. 5. Cambridge: Cambridge University Press, 1919.

Strachan, Hew. *European Armies and the Conduct of War*. London: Allen and Unwin, 1983.

Strachan, Hew. *From Waterloo to Balaclava: Tactics, Technology, and the British Army, 1815–1854*. Cambridge: Cambridge University Press, 1985.

Straub, Paul F. *Medical Service in Campaign: A Handbook for Medical Officers in the Field*. Philadelphia: Blakiston, 1910.

Strong, William E. *A Trip to the Yellowstone National Park, in July, August, and September, 1875*. Washington, D.C.: n.p., 1876.

Sullivan, Reginald N. *"Somewhere in France," Personal Letters of Reginald Noel Sullivan S.S.U. 65 of the American Ambulance Field Service*. San Francisco: Printed for Private Circulation, 1917.

Thurstan, Violetta. *Field Hospital and Flying Column; Being the Journal of an English Nursing Sister in Belgium and Russia*. New York: Putnam, 1915.

Tiffany, Francis. *Life of Dorothea Dix*. Boston: Houghton Mifflin, 1890.

Tobey, James A. *The Medical Department of the Army: Its History, Activities and Organization*. Baltimore: Johns Hopkins University Press, 1927.

Toland, Edward D. *The Aftermath of Battle: With the Red Cross in France*. New York: Macmillan, 1916.

Toulmin, Colonel Harry, Jr. *With Pershing in Mexico*. Harrisburg, Pennsylvania: Military Service, 1935.

Trask, David F. *The War with Spain in 1898*. New York: Macmillan, 1981.

Tripler, Charles Stuart. *Handbook for the Military Surgeon: Being a Compendium of the Duties of the Medical Officer in the Field*. 2d ed.; Cincinnati: Robert Clarke, 1861.

Tripler, Charles Stuart. *Manual of the Medical Officer of the Army of the United States, Part I: Recruiting and Inspection of Recruits*. Cincinnati: Wrightson, 1858.

Tunis, Edwin. *Wheels: A Pictorial History*. New York: World Publications, 1955.

United States Government. *Description of the Models of Hospital Steam Vessels*. Philadelphia: n.p., 1876.

United States Government. *International Exhibition of 1876. Hospital of Medical Department, United States Army. Description of the Models of Hospital Cars*. Washington, D.C.: Government Printing Office, 1876.

United States Government. *World's Columbian Exposition, Chicago, Illinois, 1892–93. War Department Exhibit. Medical Department, United States Army. Description of the Models of Hospital Cars from the Army Medical Museum, Washington, D.C.* Chicago: n.p., 1893.

United States Government. Army Chemical Corps. *A Comparative Study of World War Casualties from Gas and Other Weapons*. Prepared by H. L. Gilchrist. Washington, D.C.: Government Printing Office, 1928.

United States Government. Army War College. *Motor Transport in Campaign*. Washington, D.C.: Government Printing Office, 1916.

United States Government. Medical Department, U.S. Army. *Exhibit, Class 3, No. 3. Description of the Models of Hospital Cars, from the United States Army Medical Museum, Washington, D.C.* New Orleans: n.p., 1884–85.

United States Government. Military Commission to Europe, 1855–1856. *The Armies of Europe: Comprising Descriptions in Detail of the Military Systems of England, France, Russia, Prussia, Austria, and Sardinia, Adapting Their Advantages to All Arms of the United States Service*. Philadelphia:Lippincott, 1861.

United States Government. Surgeon General's Office. *Circular No. 1. Instructions for Folding Litter for Transportation of Sick and Wounded in Absence of Litters*. Washington, D.C.: Government Printing Office, 1901.

United States Government. Surgeon General's Office. *The Medical and Surgical History of the War of the Rebellion (1861–65). Prepared, in Accordance with the Acts of Congress, under the Direction of Surgeon General Joseph K. Barnes, United States Army*. 3 parts in 6 vols.; Washington, D.C.: Government Printing Office, 1870–88.

United States Government. Surgeon General's Office. *Statistical Report on the Sickness and Mortality in the Army of the United States*. Washington, D.C.: J. Gideon, Jr., 1840–60.

United States Government. War Department. *Annual Reports*. Washington, D.C.: Government Printing Office.

United States Government. War Department. *Revised Regulations for the Army of the United States, 1861*. Philadelphia: George W. Childs, 1862.

United States Government. War Department. *The War of the Rebellion: A Compilation of the Official Records of the Union and Confederate Armies*. 4 series, 130 vols.; Washington, D.C.: Government Printing Office, 1880–1901.

United States Sanitary Commission. *The Sanitary Commission of the United States Army: A Succinct Narrative of Its Works and Purposes*. New York: Arno Press, 1972 [1864].

Upton, Emory. *The Armies of Asia and Europe: Embracing Official Reports on the Armies of Japan, China, India, Persia, Italy, Russia, Austria, Germany, France, and England*. New York: Appleton, 1878.

Upton, Emory. *The Military Policy of the United States*. Washington, D.C.: Government Printing Office, 1904.

Upton, Emory. *A New System of Infantry Tactics, Double and Single Rank, Adopted to American Topography and Improved Fire-Arms*. New York: Appleton, 1873.

Van Creveld, Martin L. *Supplying War: Logistics from Wallenstein to Patton*. Cambridge: Cambridge University Press, 1977.

Vanderveen, Bart H. *The Observer's Army Vehicles Directory to 1940*. New York: Frederick Warne, 1974.

Vedder, Edward B. *The Medical Aspects of Chemical Warfare*. Baltimore: Williams and Wilkins, 1925.

Vedder, Edward B. *Sanitation for Medical Officers*. Philadelphia: Lea and Febiger, 1917.

Vess, David M. *Medical Revolution in France, 1789–1796*. Gainesville: University Presses of Florida, 1975.

Wagner, Arthur L. *Campaign of Königgrätz: A Study of the Austro-Prussian Conflict in the Light of the American Civil War*. Westport, Connecticut: Greenwood Press, 1972 [1889].

Wagner, Arthur L. *Organization and Tactics*. London: B. Westerman, 1895.

Wagner, Arthur L. *The Service of Security and Information*. Washington, D.C.: J. J. Chapman, 1893.

Warner, Philip. *The Crimean War: A Reappraisal*. London: Barker, 1972.

Watson, William. *Letters of a Civil War Surgeon*. Lafayette, Indiana: Purdue University Research Foundation, 1961.

Weigley, Russell F. *The American Way of War: A History of United States Military Strategy and Policy*. New York: Macmillan, 1973.

Weigley, Russell F. *History of the United States Army*. New York: Macmillan, 1967.

Weigley, Russell F. *Quartermaster General of the Union Army: A Biography of M. C. Meigs*. New York: Columbia University Press, 1959.

Weigley, Russell F. *Towards an American Army: Military Thought from Washington to Marshall*. New York: Columbia University Press, 1962.

Western Sanitary Commission. *Report of the Western Sanitary Commission for the Year Ending June 1, 1863*. St. Louis: Western Sanitary Commission, 1863.

Whitman, Walt. *The Wound Dresser*. New York: Bodley Press, 1949.

Wilber, C. K. *Revolutionary Medicine, 1700–1800*. Chester, Connecticut: Globe Pequot, 1980.

Wiley, Bell Irvin. *The Life of Johnny Reb: The Common Soldier of the Confederacy*. Indianapolis: Bobbs-Merrill, 1943.

Wiley, Bell Irvin. *They Who Fought Here*. New York: Macmillan, 1959.

Willard, DeForest. *Ambulance Service in Philadelphia*. Philadelphia: n.p., 1883.

Winter, Denis. *Death's Men: Soldiers of the Great War*. London: Allen Lane, 1978.

Winternitz, M. C. *Collected Studies on the Pathology of War Gas Poisoning*. New Haven, Connecticut: Yale University Press, 1920.

Woodham-Smith, Cecil. *Florence Nightingale, 1820–1910*. London: Constable, 1950.

Wyatt, Horace. *Motor Transports in War*. London: Hodder and Stoughton, 1914.

Zahn, Carl. *Uber Lazarethzuge*. Neustadt: D. Kranzbühler, 1871.

Zavodovsky, A. *Transport spécial des malades et des blessés en temps de guerre par voies ferrées*. Saint Petersburg: n.p., 1874.

Zimmerman, Leo M., and Ilza Veith. *Great Ideas in the History of Surgery*. Baltimore: Williams and Wilkins, 1961.

Zouche Marshall, J. J. de. *Stretcher Drill*. London: J. and A. Churchill, 1904.

Index

Medical Humanities Series

Glen W. Davidson, Editor

The Medical Humanities Series is devoted to publication of original or out-of-print materials relating to perceptions the humanities bring to clinical practice and health care. In this way the series also serves to promote communication among clinicians, humanists, and the general public.

Several titles in the series have been commissioned for areas in which little material is available. The following disciplines are represented in the series: anthropology, decision making in medicine, history, jurisprudence, literature, philosophy, religious studies, rhetoric, and visual arts. Unsolicited manuscripts will be considered.

The series is a project of the Department of Medical Humanities at Southern Illinois University School of Medicine in Springfield.

John S. Haller, Jr., holds a dual appointment as professor of history at Southern Illinois University at Carbondale and professor of medical humanities at the SIU School of Medicine. He is author of *Outcasts from Evolution: Scientific Attitudes of Racial Inferiority, 1859–1900* (winner of the Anisfield-Wolf Prize in Race Relations); *The Physician and Sexuality in Victorian America* (with Robin M. Haller); *American Medicine in Transition, 1840–1910*; and *Medical Protestants: The Eclectics in American Medicine, 1825–1939* (forthcoming), as well as numerous articles on the history of nineteenth-century sexuality, anthropology, medicine, and pharmacy.

3/94 6   7/05 9